Natural
Compresses
& Poultices

"Ancient Chinese physicians believed that a competent healer had no need to cut into the body; herbal poultices, acupuncture, water treatments, and herbal brews were the mark of the advanced practitioner. In this book, we are given a glimpse of modern cures that do not involve violence to the physical form. With simple and easy-to-follow directions, Dr. Vasey shows us how to use the skin, our largest organ of elimination, to effect a cure. This book includes many commonsense precautions and a well-crafted collection of compresses and applications for common injuries and conditions, many of which involve foods we already have in the kitchen like potatoes, onions, and lemons. I highly recommend this book!"

ELLEN EVERT HOPMAN, AUTHOR OF
SECRET MEDICINES FROM YOUR GARDEN AND
A DRUID'S HERBAL OF SACRED TREE MEDICINE

Natural Compresses & Poultices

Safe and Simple Folk Medicine Treatments for 70 Common Conditions

CHRISTOPHER VASEY, N.D.

Translated by Jon E. Graham

Healing Arts Press
Rochester, Vermont

Healing Arts Press
One Park Street
Rochester, Vermont 05767
www.HealingArtsPress.com

Healing Arts Press is a division of Inner Traditions International

Originally published in French under the title *Compresses et cataplasmes: Les remèdes miracles (et bon marché) de nos ancêtres* by Éditions Jouvence, www.editions-jouvence.com, info@editions-jouvence.com
First U.S. edition published in 2019 by Healing Arts Press

Note to the reader: This book is intended as an informational guide. The remedies, approaches, and techniques described herein are meant to supplement, and not to be a substitute for, professional medical care or treatment. They should not be used to treat a serious ailment without prior consultation with a qualified health care professional.

Cataloging-in-Publication Data for this title is available from the Library of Congress

ISBN 978-1-62055-737-2 (print)
ISBN 978-1-62055-738-9 (ebook)

Printed and bound in the United States by McNaughton & Gunn, Inc.

10 9 8 7 6 5 4 3 2 1

Text design and layout by Virginia Scott Bowman
This book was typeset in Garamond Premier Pro with Gill Sans and Berkeley Oldstyle used as display typefaces
Illustration on page 8 © Neokryuger/Stockfresh; illustrations on pages 15–17 by Jean Augagneur

To send correspondence to the author of this book, mail a first-class letter to the author c/o Inner Traditions • Bear & Company, One Park Street, Rochester, VT 05767, and we will forward the communication, or contact the author directly at **www.christophervasey.ch.**

Contents

Rapid Relief with Easy Home Remedies

When suffering from headache, toothache, indigestion, sinusitis, painful menstrual periods, joint inflammation, nerve pain, cough, and so on, the patient's primary desire—even before that of being cured—is to find rapid relief from pain and suffering.

What is the most effective nonpharmaceutical way for someone who is not a health care professional to do this?

A simple method that can easily be done by anyone, often using materials you already have on hand, is to use compresses and poultices. When applied to the ailing part of the body, a compress or poultice can make the patient feel better immediately. It can soothe pain, reduce swelling of inflamed tissues, relax the patient, and take an active role in the healing process. Applying one of these remedies is extremely easy, and the necessary ingredients and materials (scraps of cloth, onions, potatoes, and so forth) are readily available. Rapid relief can therefore be easily and quickly achieved in all circumstances, even if no professional health practitioner or prescription is available.

Compresses and poultices are not only useful for first aid,

they also provide valuable treatments for existing illnesses, whether chronic or acute.

But we would be mistaken to believe that compresses and poultices can cure all disorders. While it is true that in certain cases they represent the most appropriate treatment, in other instances they are at best a backup or complementary treatment. In these cases their use will not be sufficient to adequately treat the condition.

If compresses and poultices were highly valued by our grandmothers and the traditional medical practices of many countries through the centuries, it is because they provide a healing method that is simple, quick, and effective. In addition—and this should not be underestimated in our modern times—they offer natural and nontoxic methods for healing.

1

Why Are Compresses and Poultices So Effective?

Elimination Equals Healing

Illness is due to an accumulation of toxins in the body's physiological cellular terrain. Healing is achieved through the elimination of these toxins by means of the body's emunctory, or excretory, organs. The skin is one of these organs of waste clearance, and it is where compresses and poultices go to work.

There is something disconcerting about the use of compresses and poultices. How is it that simple applications of cloth steeped in hot or cold water, or applications of clay, potato, or cottage cheese, can have an effect that is not only therapeutic but also powerfully beneficial?

The fact remains that there are proven results over a number of centuries. If compresses and poultices had not been used successfully by the great physicians of antiquity (Hippocrates, Galen, and so on) and, until the early twentieth century, in all hospitals, and if they were not still being used successfully in the folk medicine of the vast majority of developing countries

3

and in the West, they would by no means be considered serious procedures and their effectiveness would be rejected as a myth.

📚 A Little History

Hippocrates, often referred to as the Father of Medicine, was a Greek physician who lived during the fifth century BCE. His enduring legacy is a vast body of knowledge on the art of healing that is still relevant today. His approach was quite naturopathic: do no harm, treat causes and not symptoms, and stress the importance of diet.

Their efficacy is quite authentic. However, their use requires an understanding of the true nature of disease and of the functions of the skin, as well as what compresses and poultices are and what effects they can trigger in the body when applied to the skin.

📚 A Little History

Galen, dubbed the Prince of Medicine, practiced in Rome during the second century CE. He brilliantly synthesized all of the known medical practices through his time and gave new impetus to the art of healing. This included a more extensive study of anatomy and experimental research. His influence on Eastern medicine lasted into the seventeenth century.

WHAT IS A DISEASE?

Illness is not an independent, self-contained entity that enters our bodies from the outside. Illness is simply a defective state of our organs and their functions. From the perspective of natural medicine, illnesses are not created by chance but are always the result of the deterioration of our inner environment, or "physiological terrain."

Our terrain consists of all of our bodily fluids: blood, lymph, and the cellular fluids in which all our cells and organs are immersed, which simultaneously serve as their source of nourishment and their environment. As long as the terrain maintains its proper characteristics, our cells function normally and our organs remain in good health. When this is no longer the case and the composition of our bodily fluids has been altered, cellular life is disrupted, the organs become sick, and germs can develop and infect the body.

Thus we can see that illness is not possible unless the terrain has been damaged.

WHAT CAUSES THIS BREAKDOWN OF THE TERRAIN?

This damage can occur in two different ways, which can combine and accumulate. On the one hand, the cellular terrain can become saturated with metabolic wastes (toxins) or poisons from the outside; this creates overload diseases. On the other hand, the terrain can develop a deficiency of substances needed by the cells (amino acids, vitamins, minerals), which will lead to deficiency diseases.

When they collect in the body, toxins thicken blood, clog blood vessels, cause congestion in the organs, and weaken the body's resistance to infection. Any deficiencies in needed substances will only increase the poisoned state of the body, because organs deprived of the nutrients they need function less efficiently. This will result in increased production of wastes, which will eventually saturate the terrain.

☞ Good to Know

The terrain: The human body is 70 percent liquid, including intracellular fluid (50 percent), extracellular fluid and lymph (15 percent), and blood (5 percent).

The root cause of the vast majority of physical disorders and diseases is an undesirable accumulation of waste, including cholesterol that causes blood to thicken, fatty deposits that hamper circulation, "crystals" that block and inflame joints, acids that injure the skin of eczema sufferers, pus that oozes from abscesses, stones that hinder the work of the gallbladder, phlegm that burdens the bronchia and sinuses, and so on.

CLEANSING THE TERRAIN

Because this accumulated waste causes so many disorders, the first objective of the health practitioner must be to try to rid the body of the toxins clogging the various tissues. There are five possible avenues for eliminating waste: the liver, intestines, kidneys, lungs, and skin.* Of these, the skin is the field of activity for compresses and poultices. In contrast to all of the other emunctory organs, each of which specializes in the elimination of a specific kind of waste, the skin is capable of discharging every variety of toxin and poison, which is why therapeutic approaches that focus on the skin and use compresses and poultices are highly effective.

---

*For more on this see my book *Optimal Detox* (Healing Arts Press, 2013).

2

The Skin and Its Functions

Filtration and Excretion

The skin has the ability to eliminate every kind of toxin or poison. Moreover, it has multiple functions that support this elimination.

The skin is not simply a protective shell that contains all the body's tissues. It is an independent organ, with many often-unrecognized functions that benefit from compresses and poultices.

THE VASCULAR FUNCTION OF THE SKIN

The skin is irrigated by a finely developed network of blood capillaries. Capillaries are extremely slender blood vessels (as fine as hairs) that penetrate into the depths of the tissues and carry oxygen and nutritive substances. They also carry out wastes that are expelled by the cells.

Capillaries have the ability to dilate enormously, doubling or tripling in diameter. They also have the ability to contract so much that their diameter becomes too narrow to allow the passage of red blood corpuscles.

☞ Good to Know

A significant portion of the body's blood supply can be found in the capillaries of the skin. When dilated, they can hold up to 20 percent of the total mass of blood in the human body.

Thanks to the application of compresses and poultices, it is possible to draw a considerable quantity of blood toward the skin or send it in the opposite direction, toward the deeper organs, depending on whether the compresses or poultices used are hot or cold. This property is exceedingly valuable because blood plays a primordial role in providing nutrition and oxygenizing the cells, and it is a vital player in all of the body's defense processes.

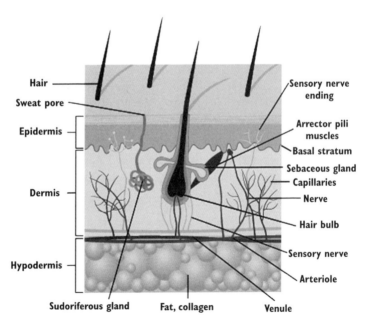

Anatomy of the skin

THE MUSCULAR
FUNCTION OF THE SKIN

The muscles contained within the skin are quite small, of course, but they are also quite numerous. When all of them contract at the same time, their effect on blood circulation, the production of heat and perspiration, and cellular exchanges is tremendous.

There are three kinds of muscles in the skin:

1. Tiny *arrector pili* muscles attached to hair follicles. When someone feels cold or very frightened, the arrector pili muscles contract and make "goose bumps" that cause the hairs to "stand on end," thus shutting the pores and trapping as much air as possible to prevent loss of body heat.
2. Muscles contained in the walls of the capillaries. Their role is to accommodate the vasodilation and vasoconstriction of these extremely fine blood vessels.
3. Smooth fibers isolated inside the cutaneous tissue. They provide the skin with the elasticity and tone it needs to handle the various demands and hazards to which it is subject.

THE ELIMINATORY
FUNCTION OF THE SKIN

The skin has several different paths for fulfilling its function of eliminating wastes from the body.

The Sudoriferous Glands

Numbering around two million (210 to 650 per square inch of skin), the sudoriferous glands expel sweat through the pores of the body. Unlike other glands, they do not produce anything.

Their only responsibility is to extract fluid charged with toxic substances from the bloodstream, which they then eliminate in the form of sweat.

The sudoriferous glands function in almost the same way as the nephrons, which are the functional units of the kidneys, and can be considered a kind of third kidney that is dispersed across the entire surface of the body. Likewise, the wastes eliminated by the sudoriferous glands are similar in nature to those eliminated by the kidneys. These are water-soluble wastes, such as depleted minerals (phosphorus and so on), protein wastes (urea, uric acid, creatine), acids (lactic acid), and chemical residue from pharmaceutical medications and pollution.

The sudoriferous glands' filtration of wastes and poisons is dependent on blood flow, which is almost nonexistent when the body is cold and the blood retreats from the skin's surface. Conversely, blood flow is quite considerable when the body is warm; the capillaries fill with blood and it circulates quickly. An easy way to increase the speed of localized blood circulation is to use compresses and poultices.

The Sebaceous Glands

The sebaceous glands are located at the roots of the hair follicles. There are roughly three hundred thousand of these glands on the total surface of the body. They filter the blood transported to them via the blood capillaries and rid it of the nearly insoluble wastes it contains. These wastes include carbohydrates, fats, mucus, dead germ cells, and various substances that are toxic to the body, such as mercury and iodine.

The wastes are expelled into the sebum, an oily substance that helps lubricate the skin. When a sebaceous gland becomes clogged, the plugged sebum darkens due to oxidation and appears as a "blackhead." If the gland becomes too congested to shed dead cells, a pimple forms with a white head.

The nature of the wastes expelled by the sebaceous glands makes these glands comparable to tiny versions of the liver scattered across the skin.

The Basal Stratum (The Malpighian Layer)

The basal stratum forms the third path for cutaneous elimination, which is the outermost layer of the skin. There is still much to learn about this layer, but studies have shown that it possesses around seventy enzymes that break down cellular and microbial debris, as well as any toxins that reach its level.

Once these waste products have been broken down into simpler particles, the helpful substances are deposited back into the bloodstream, where they can be used by the body. The unwanted substances that remain after this selection process are directed toward the skin surface to be eliminated from the body.

This elimination takes place using a well-known process. The toxic substance is neutralized within a cell by sulfur (keratinization). Following this step, the cell expels its core and the fluid it contains and then flattens and dehydrates. It then gradually rises toward the most superficial layers of the skin, where it finally separates from the body in the form of tiny flakes of dried skin (exfoliation).

THE ASSIMILATORY FUNCTION OF THE SKIN

The skin is not merely an excretory organ; it is also an organ of assimilation that is capable of absorbing some of the substances that come into contact with its most superficial layers.

Studies have shown that the skin assimilates mineral salts found in thermal spring water. Similarly, medicinal and moisturizing creams and skin-enhancing cosmetic products would have no effect if the skin were not capable of absorbing their active ingredients.

The assimilatory function of the skin is used to its best effect with the application of poultices, such as clay poultices that restore minerals to the body and cabbage leaf poultices that regenerate and heal.

THE NERVE FUNCTION OF THE SKIN

There is a finely developed network of nerve endings in the skin. Originating in the central nervous system, these nerve endings branch out comprehensively in the epidermis and record even the tiniest stimulations that come from outside the body.

There are four different kinds of sensory receptors, each specializing in a specific kind of sensation. They are the receptors of contact, pressure, vibration, and temperature.

The skin is not satisfied with simply hosting and protecting this hypersensitive network of nerves but also reacts to the signals it sends. For example, the sensations of hot and cold will cause the pores of the skin to open or close, circulation to accelerate or abate, chemical reactions to increase or diminish, and so forth. These transformations of the skin's metabolism can be used advantageously and deliberately by the application of compresses and poultices.

3

Compresses and Poultices

Natural Healing with Cloth Wraps,
Medicinal Plants, Vegetables, and Earth

Compresses are pieces of cloth that have been soaked in water or other liquids. Poultices are cohesive preparations of mineral or plant origin.

COMPRESSES

A compress is a piece of cloth that has been saturated with water and then folded several times so that it can be placed over the ailing part of the body. Fabrics used for this purpose are made from natural fibers, such as linen or cotton. Synthetic fabric should never be used. The temperature of the water in which the compress is soaked before it is applied can vary greatly depending on the desired results of this therapy. It can be freezing, cold (68°F or below), cool, lukewarm, body temperature, or hot (up to 113°F). A compress will be forcefully or only slightly wrung out, allowing it to retain the desired amount of water. On exceptional occasions, the compress will be applied completely dry (dry-wrapped).

The size and surface area of a compress depends on which part of the body is being treated. It will be small if it is applied to dress a finger, but for treating a fever, for example, it can cover the entire torso.

The liquid used to moisten compresses is most often water, but infusions or decoctions of medicinal plants can also be used, or vinegar or whey mixed with water.

Once it has been placed on the ailing part of the body, a compress is almost always covered. It can be covered by a protective cloth to prevent moisture from dampening the patient's clothing, bed, or anything else in the immediate vicinity, or a wool cloth can be used to keep the compress from cooling down too quickly.

WHAT FABRICS ARE
BEST FOR THIS PURPOSE?

In order to give the reader the broadest latitude in the choice of fabric, I am going to use the neutral term of "cloth" in the instructions without offering any more details. Ideally the primary cloth (the one that will be soaked in liquid) should be made of linen, the second cloth that covers it or is used to cover a poultice should be cotton, and the third one that covers both the other cloths should be entirely wool. Ideally again, the size of each cloth should be increasingly larger than the one it is covering, the first being 1 to 1½ inches smaller than the second, which itself will be 1 to 1½ inches smaller than the third cloth.

However, equally effective compresses can be made as needed from the many different fabrics found in today's average home. They simply need to be cut or folded to the desired

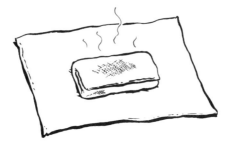

The hot compress is placed on top of a kitchen cloth.

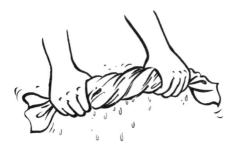

Wringing out the compress

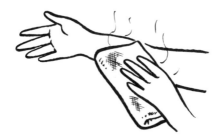

Monitoring the temperature

dimensions. These might include dish towels and kitchen cloths, bath towels, washcloths, strips of old sheets, pillowcases, tablecloths, shirts, diapers, and so on. Only synthetic fabrics must be avoided.

One practical method for settling once and for all the cloth issue is to buy lengths of the necessary fabrics (linen, cotton, wool) that are commercially manufactured by some companies for the express purpose of making compresses.

POULTICES

Poultices are paste-like preparations that are sometimes applied directly to the skin and sometimes first wrapped in a thin cloth. Poultices are made from a vast array of different materials, such as ice cubes, earth substances (clay or volcanic soil), medicinal plants (birch leaves, seaweed, and the like), vegeta-

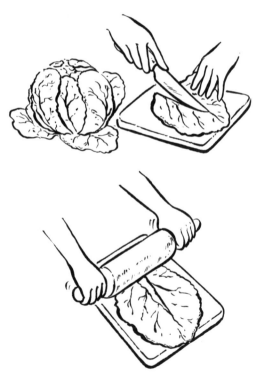

Cabbage poultice: remove the center stalk,
then crush the leaves with a rolling pin.

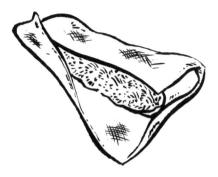

Flaxseed poultice: sealing the poultice

bles (potato, cabbage, onion, carrot), fruits (lemons, peaches, apples), seeds (flax, mustard seed, and so on), and animal by-products (beeswax, small-curd cottage cheese, Greek yogurt, and others with a similar consistency).

As is the case with compresses, poultices are applied hot or cold depending on the desired result—the physiological reactions you are seeking to trigger in both the skin and the deeper organs.

4

The Effects of Compresses and Poultices on the Skin

Rebalancing the Terrain

The many effective methods of using compresses and poultices for a variety of results make it possible to adapt treatment to appropriately address the patient and the disease.

The healing effect is created by the contact of the compresses and poultices with the skin. This action is fourfold: thermic, chemical, revulsive, and absorbent. The thermic effect is the primary therapeutic action and is critical for the healing process.

THERMIC ACTION

Once it has been applied to the body, the compress or poultice acts as a "second skin." However, this additional layer is not the same temperature as the actual skin and therefore creates a thermic imbalance in the body.

The body is not able to tolerate the temperature change of its tissues for a very long period because it endangers the survival of the cells and the proper functioning of physiological activity. This thermic imbalance therefore forces the body to make an effort to restore its equilibrium, and it is the various physiological processes it sets in motion to achieve this goal that form the basis of the healing action of compresses and poultices.

The thermic imbalance will be more significant when the temperature of the application is much higher or lower than the temperature of the body. The possibility of restoring equilibrium is quite promising for temperatures falling between 68°F and 104°F. Beyond that range—for example, a compress as hot as 113°F, an ice cube poultice as cold as 32°F—a much more intense reaction is elicited from the body.

The degree of thermic imbalance will also be determined by the thickness of the poultice or the amount of liquid in the compress. Because there is greater density, the thicker this "second skin" is, the more the body will have to struggle to restore normal body temperature. While a thin piece of cold, wrung-out cloth is quickly warmed by the body, the same cannot be said about a compress consisting of five or six layers of cloth saturated with ice water.

The surface area of the compress or poultice is also an important factor because covering a greater area affects a larger portion of the body and will demand greater effort to restore the ideal skin temperature.

☞ Good to Know

Compresses and poultices cause a different reaction in the body depending on whether the application is hot or cold. Their healing effect essentially results from the body's physiological reactions to a thermic imbalance.

Another decisive factor is the length of time the application remains on the skin. The longer the application causing the body to go out of balance remains in contact with the body, the harder it must struggle to restore that balance.

Cold Applications

The reaction to a cold application goes through two stages. In the first phase the body tightens its tissues to the maximum extent possible in an effort to create a barrier against the attack of the cold temperature. The capillaries in the skin take part in this reaction by contracting and thus forcing the blood they contain into the deeper tissues. This means that cutaneous circulation is brought almost to a complete halt. But the absence of the blood that provides the cells with oxygen and fuels the skin will cause a general slowdown in the functions of cellular metabolism: nutrition, oxygenation, combustion, and elimination.

This first stage is of short duration. The body must react very quickly to restore the proper level of heat to the cutaneous tissues and strive to change the temperature of the source of the cold that is causing it difficulties, meaning the compress or poultice.

This is where the second stage begins. The reaction of withdrawal is replaced by a phase that goes in the other direction. Massive amounts of blood are drawn into the skin's blood capillary network so that it is available for the heat borrowed from the depths of the body. The capillaries dilate when they fill with this blood. Circulation of warm blood becomes rapid and intense, constantly replacing the blood that has lost its heat in the skin. Now the cells again begin receiving the oxygen and nutrients they need to function properly. Cellular life, which was momentarily dormant, revives and soon adopts the highly elevated rhythm that has been initiated by the reaction of the body's defenses. Because of the attack of cold, this metabolic speed is higher than normal and makes it possible to make up for the delay to some extent.

The healing effect is caused by the fact that the ailing cells are now better oxygenated and nourished, but also because they are now rid of the toxins that caused the disease. Furthermore, the intensification of circulation and cellular exchanges facilitates the access of lymphocytes from the immune system and of healing substances from the glands (anti-inflammatory substances, hormones, and so on) to the ailing area.

Warm Applications

The body's reactions do not go through the first stage that is described in the previous section (contraction caused by the cold), but thanks to the delivery of heat, they go straight to the second stage of cutaneous metabolic reactions. The strength of this acceleration is directly proportionate to the degree of heat applied. It requires only a small amount of energy from the body because the heat is not produced by the body, as is the case with the cold applications, but delivered from outside by the hot compress or poultice.

When Should Hot or Cold Be Used?

Hot and warm applications require only a small amount of reactive energy from the patient's body, which makes them very appropriate for people with low vitality or who have been weakened by illness or age. Because of their properties, hot applications are recommended for warming chilled regions (cold extremities, degenerative arthritis), loosening areas that are stiff (frozen joints) or contracted (spasms), and accelerating the sluggish (reduced circulation, sluggish system).

👆 **Good to Know**

Generally speaking, cold (short) is more often used for inflammation and acute disorders, whereas heat is recommended for chronic problems. But there are exceptions (see the practical portion of the book, chapter 5).

Oddly enough, applications that are long and cold have the same effect as hot applications. Indeed, the body is actually more than capable of reheating tissues that have been attacked by the cold. This process takes a certain amount of time to manifest, but once it is established, it is much more intense because it has been actively produced by the body itself. Given the fact that it requires sufficient energy reserves to confront the cold, these long, cold applications are only recommended for individuals who have high vitality.

In contrast, short cold applications have the opposite effect. The cold chills what is hot (soothes inflammation), causes what is dilated to contract (unblocks congested tissues), slows what has accelerated (hyperfunctioning glandular or other system), gives tone to the soft (slack tissues and sluggish system), and calms pain (anesthetic effect).

CHEMICAL ACTION

The therapeutic success of compresses and poultices can also be attributed to the assimilatory capacity of the skin.

The skin has the ability to absorb substances that are useful to the body, substances that are contained in the materials used to make compresses and poultices. These include vitamins and minerals provided by the fruits, vegetables, and clay; active properties of medicinal plants; the softening substances offered by flaxseed mucilage; the disinfectant properties of onions; and so forth.

In the majority of cases the joint action of temperature combined with the properties of the material are responsible for the healing effect. Applications in which only the action of the nutritive or medicinal substance comes into play are rare. One example is arnica compresses used for bruises or sprains.

REVULSIVE ACTION

Certain substances, such as mustard, have an irritating effect on the skin. If they are left in contact with it for an extended period of time, they will cause a painful inflammation. Initially there will be a minor stinging sensation that will gradually start to burn. The skin will become red, blisters will appear, and finally an open wound can form if the application is left on for too long.

Of course, when they are used in compresses and poultices, revulsive substances are not intended to injure the skin but to artificially trigger a healing process. The way it works is the skin, wanting to defend itself when confronted by this attack, draws a large amount of blood into itself. The purpose of this influx is to better irrigate the tissues so that irritating substances can be neutralized and expelled from the body more easily, and to facilitate the repair of lesions.

The duration of a skin application for a revulsive compress or poultice is therefore quite short. It must be long enough for the attack to be felt by the body and the defensive process set into motion, but not so long that the irritation actually becomes an injury. These applications that require sensitive handling are worth the extra attention as they make it possible to quickly direct an intensified healing process to a given part of the body. The effects are not restricted to the surface but reach the depths of the body. As the surface tissues become congested with the influx of blood, the deep tissues become decongested. The blood leaves the depths and rises toward the skin, carrying the toxins that will be easily eliminated by the skin once they reach the surface.

Revulsive compresses and poultices are used to treat poorly irrigated deep tissues, such as painful joints (arthritis, rheumatism), or to bring rapid relief to an organ encumbered by wastes. One example would be the bronchia in the event of asthma.

ABSORBENT ACTION

Two poultices are exceptional for their powerful properties of absorption and suction. These poultices are made from clay or cabbage leaves.

Clay and Cabbage Leaf Poultices

There is a wealth of supporting evidence for the ability of clay and cabbage leaf to extract and expel substances from the body. The primary target of this capacity appears to be toxins that are lying stagnant in the tissues, and not useful vitamins and minerals. The suction action takes place through the entire thickness of the skin, into the deepest layers of tissue. The metabolic residues and wastes removed from the cells in this way then travel through the tissue layers separating them from the surface of the body and finally through the skin without harming it.

🖐 Good to Know

Dr. Jean Valnet, a pioneering researcher in natural healing, noted that cabbage appears to have a particular affinity for the contaminated "humors," as he called them, that it compels to leave the tissues. It even seems that its application to restricted points of a widespread disorder are beneficial in treating the entire disorder. The far-flung toxins appear to be attracted to the cabbage.

In an extended course of treatment, repeated applications are necessary because the initial poultices will cleanse only superficial tissues. However, once those tissues have been purged of their wastes, the way is clear for debris that lies deeper in the body to exit. These wastes will then gradually rise to the surface for removal. By leaving the tissues, they allow for the regeneration and healing of the diseased organs.

The properties of suction and absorption possessed by clay and cabbage poultices work regardless of their temperature. But when temperature is also a factor, as is the case with clay poultices that can be applied either hot or cold, the stimulating and eliminating properties of heat will then combine with the suction action of the clay.

The most obvious use of these kinds of poultices is for cleansing the skin: pimples, cuts, abscesses, varicose ulcers, and so forth. In these cases the applications are renewed fairly often to avoid auto-poisoning, as the mass of pus and mucus that is extracted will quickly saturate the poultice. When they become permeated by these wastes, cabbage leaves, for example, are sometimes completely "rotted" and "cooked" by their presence, which can easily be observed when replacing the old poultice with a fresh one.

HOW DO THE EFFECTS OF COMPRESSES AND POULTICES REACH THE BODY'S INTERNAL ORGANS?

The skin is an extremely thin organ with a thickness that varies from 0.12 millimeter at the eyelids to around 2 millimeters on the palm of the hand, where it is thicker in order to resist the numerous demands placed there. This thinness explains why the effects of compresses and poultices inevitably infiltrate the underlying tissues. This is how an acceleration of blood flow in the outer layers of the body automatically triggers an increase in the rate of circulation in the surrounding tissues covered by the poultice or compress, as the blood carried by the vessels comes from these deeper tissues. The same holds true for the intensification of metabolic activities, whose speed is progressively transmitted to the surrounding tissues, where the metabolic rates will also increase.

As stated earlier, once the superficial tissue layers have been freed of the wastes burdening them, the way is clear for wastes in the lower layers to percolate to the surface to be eliminated. This phenomenon is repeated from one layer to the next until the deep organs are finally reached and are then able to rid themselves of the toxic waste that has made them sick.

An in-depth effect is, of course, only possible if the action of the compresses and poultices is fairly sustained, which depends on their temperature, their density, and the frequency with which they are applied.

5

The Application of Compresses and Poultices

Examples and Recommendations from Head to Toe

To help you move from theory into practice, here are concrete examples of the application of compresses and/or poultices for more than seventy health disorders.

Nothing could be simpler than putting together a compress or poultice. What is much less simple, which can sometimes be a challenge, is the correct application for a specific problem.

In this kind of disorder, should this compress or that poultice be used? Is a cold application advisable, or the opposite, a warm one? What is the precise location for each application? How often should the compress be changed? These are some of the questions that undoubtedly occur to anyone working with an unfamiliar healing modality.

Fortunately, these are remedies of great simplicity, which we know because our ancestors fashioned them in much more primitive circumstances than we are lucky enough to have today.

The purpose of this book is to make the use of compresses

and poultices highly accessible and eliminate all possible obstacles concerning the choice of procedure and the modalities of application. Therefore, for every disease covered, this book will provide instruction on not only two or three of the most appropriate compresses and poultices but also the materials necessary to create them, the way to prepare and apply them, and the length of the application and how often it should be changed.

✗ Tips and Tricks

The patient's feeling of well-being or distress is a valuable guide to making the applications as effective as possible.

Even a beginner can start right away. With experience and more extensive knowledge of the guiding principles of the art of healing with compresses and poultices, knowledge is increased and refined, and the practitioner is soon able to innovate and vary applications to better adapt them to each individual case.

Common sense and logic should govern the use of compresses and poultices. The instructions provided are not hard and fast rules but guidelines. They can, and should, be altered and adapted to different situations and different cases.

The Head

BUMP ON THE HEAD FOLLOWING A BLOW (GOOSE EGG)

When you crack your head against the wall, a piece of furniture, or another person, a characteristic swelling (bump) will appear at the place of impact. Applying cold to the bump will soothe the pain and, by stimulating circulation, reduce the swelling.

Ice Cube Poultice

2 or 3 ice cubes

1 ziplock plastic bag

1 protective cloth

Preparation: Place the ice cubes in the plastic bag and seal it. Wrap the bag once in the protective cloth.

Application: Place the poultice directly on the painful area.

Duration: Leave in place for as long as the calming effect is pleasant and lasting (five to fifteen minutes).

Frequency: As a general rule, one application should be enough.

HEADACHE

Headaches have a varied number of causes but occur in only two primary forms: headaches due to circulation problems, and headaches due to tension in the suboccipital muscles in the nape of the neck. These latter headaches generally have their origin in tight muscles (poor posture) and a nervous condition (stress, worry, anxiety).

Headache Caused by Dilated Blood Vessels

In the "circulatory" headache, the blood vessels that irrigate the brain are severely dilated, which provokes a painful feeling of congestion in the head. A supply of cold is therefore indicated because it will cause the blood vessels to contract back to their normal diameter, thereby encouraging better cerebral circulation.

Ice Water Compress

1 bowl of cold water

Ice cubes

1 cloth folded several times to a size that will allow
it to cover the forehead

Preparation: Place the ice cubes in the bowl of cold water. When the water is sufficiently cold, soak the compress in it amd then let some of the excess water drip off—but not too much.

Application: Place the soaked compress over the forehead.

Duration: Before it becomes warm, re-soak the compress in the freezing water and lay it back over the forehead.

Frequency: Repeat the applications as often as you like.

Variation: A second compress may be placed over the nape of the neck, either alternately or at the same time.

✚ That Little Bit Extra

As a complement to compresses on the forehead, warm poultices on the soles of the feet can prove to be quite helpful because they draw blood to the other end of the body and thereby help decongest the blood vessels in the head. The most appropriate poultices for this purpose are prepared with onions or mustard powder (see pages 104–5 for recipes and instructions).

Clay Poultice

A poultice made from clay is another option for treating this condition. See page 81 for instructions, which should be adapted for application to the forehead.

Headache Caused by Muscular Tension in the Back of the Neck

A muscular headache is engendered by prolonged contraction of the muscles of the nape of the neck and the scalp, a contraction that soon causes repercussions in the entire head. In this case warmth is called for, as it will release the tension and allow relaxation.

Hot Water Compress

Boiling water

1 cloth folded three or four times to a size large
   enough to cover the nape of the neck

1 hot water bottle filled with hot water

1 washcloth

1 kitchen towel

⚠ Caution!

The hot water bottle should be filled with hot water from the tap and not water heated on the stove, which could potentially burn the skin.

Preparation: Soak the folded cloth in the boiling water. Set it on the kitchen towel, fold the towel over it, and use the towel to wring it out. (Holding the ends, twist in opposite directions.) Wrap the wrung-out compress with a washcloth (one single thickness). This washcloth will help protect the skin from the very high temperature of the compress. The moist heat will slowly spread through it to skin level to act in a comforting and relaxing way on the taut, contracted muscles of the nape of the neck.

Application: After you have tested the temperature on the inside of your forearm, place the compress on the nape of the neck. Cover with the hot water bottle, which will help the compress maintain its heat during the entire time of its application.

Duration: Continue for ten minutes to half an hour.

Frequency: Repeat the application as many times as you like.

⚠ Caution!

Before any hot compress or poultice is placed on the body, it is important to test the temperature. It will be tolerable to other parts of the body if it can be tolerated for one minute on a part of the body that is quite sensitive to heat, such as the inner surface of the forearm.

Potato Poultice

A poultice made from hot potatoes is another option for treating this condition. See page 46 for instructions, which should be adapted for application to the nape of the neck.

MIGRAINE

A migraine is a headache confined to only one side of the head. Contrary to ordinary headaches, migraines are often accompanied by attacks of nausea, vomiting, and eye problems.

Hot Compress

1 cloth folded three or four times to a size that will
    allow it to cover the forehead and eyes

Boiling water

1 kitchen towel

Preparation: Soak the folded cloth in the boiling water. Set it on the kitchen towel, fold the towel over it, and use the towel to wring it out. (Holding the ends, twist in opposite directions.)

Application: When the compress has a tolerable temperature, which can be verified by placing it on the inside of your forearm, place it over the eyes and forehead to allow the heat to manifest its relaxing and calming effects.

Duration: Once the compress cools down, renew it by soaking it in boiling water.

Frequency: Keep renewing the compress with hot water as often as you like.

Observation: Some people subject to migraines react better to cold compresses. Proceed in the same way but soak the compress in ice water instead.

✚ That Little Bit Extra

Migraines are often accompanied by hepatic disorders. During the facial treatment of the migraine, it can be a good idea to also place a steam compress over the liver. For recipe and instructions regarding a steam compress, see page 62.

The Face
....

ACNE (PIMPLES), OILY SKIN

Acne is caused by an overabundant secretion of sebum, which is the skin's lubricant. Because of this excess production, the sebaceous glands become clogged and form a tiny swelling—a pimple—that can have a black tip (blackhead) or a white tip. It becomes red or purplish-blue because of an inflammatory reaction of the skin. Sometimes an infection accompanies the inflammation.

Clay Poultice

Healing clay powder (bentonite or other healing
   clay can be purchased via the internet, or in a
   few drugstores and big-box stores under brand
   names)

Cold water

1 wooden or glass container

1 wooden spatula to mix the water and clay together

Preparation: Mix clay with cold water until it forms a moist paste. It should be firm in consistency, not runny.

Application: Apply the clay paste to the parts of the face affected by acne. The layer applied should be a scant half-inch thick.

Duration: As it dries, the clay will extract the sebum from the sebaceous glands. Remove it once it becomes totally dry, which will be after one to two hours.

Frequency: Repeat every two to three days, depending on how well the poultice dries out the affected skin surface.

☝ Good to Know

The poultices and compresses used to treat acne all seek to decongest the sebaceous glands by sucking the sebum from them and cleansing the skin, which is often quite "oily." A healing effect is achieved by virtue of the clay; a disinfectant effect takes place thanks to medicinal plants.

Hot Compress of Medicinal Herbs

Three plants are particularly good at treating acne: echinacea and burdock for their disinfectant action, and sage for both its disinfectant action and its hormone-like properties. These properties are extremely useful during adolescence, when hormonal changes can wreak havoc with the skin.

1 cloth folded over several times to a size that will allow it to cover the affected area

Your choice of one of the following:

- **Echinacea: 50 drops of mother tincture in 1 pint of hot water**
- **Burdock decoction: Three-quarters of an ounce of root; boil for ten minutes in a pint of water. (Or 50 drops of mother tincture in 1 pint of hot water. This preparation has a more potent effect than the decoction.)**
- **Sage infusion: 1 tablespoon of sage steeped for ten minutes in a pint of hot water.**

Preparation and application: Soak the folded cloth in one of the hot preparations listed above. Drain a little of the excess liquid from the cloth, and after testing the temperature on the inside of the forearm, place it over the parts of the face requiring treatment.

Duration: Maintain for twenty to thirty minutes.

Frequency: Apply once or twice a day.

Cottage Cheese Poultice

A poultice made from small-curd cottage cheese or Greek yogurt is another option for treating this condition. See page 60 for instructions, which should be adapted for application to the face.

NEURALGIA
(FACIAL AND DENTAL)

Neuralgia is characterized by bursts of violent, stabbing pain in the jaw, teeth, ears, or temples. The pains occur on only one side and are caused by the inflammation of a sensitive nerve and the area it innervates. The recommended compresses combine the analgesic action of heat and medicinal plants.

🖐 Good to Know

Saint John's wort (*Hypericum perforatum*): This plant owes its French name, *millepertuis,* to the little translucent glands scattered over the surface of the leaves, which give them the appearance of being perforated by a thousand holes (*mille* = thousand, *pertuis* = perforations). Its English name comes from the fact that it was traditionally harvested after it flowered on Saint John's Day, June 24. These glands contain oil that has anti-inflammatory, healing, and anxiety-relieving properties.

Saint John's Wort Oil Compress

Saint John's wort oil (sold in natural food stores,
   herb shops, and some drugstores)
1 cloth handkerchief
1 wool cloth or hot water bottle
A scarf, if needed

Preparation: Pour 10 to 20 drops of Saint John's wort oil onto a handkerchief that has been folded over three or four times.

Application: Lay the compress on top of the entire area where the pain is being experienced. To heat it and maintain this heat, cover it with a wool cloth or a hot water bottle that is not very full.

Duration: Maintain for one hour at minimum or all night long. In the latter case, the compress must be fixed in place with the help of a scarf.

Frequency: Change or refresh the compress as frequently as desired.

SINUSITIS

The cheekbones and bones in the arch of the eyebrow are laced with cavities—the sinuses—that connect with the nose. Normally these cavities hold nothing but air, but under certain circumstances they can become filled with phlegm from the nasal canal. This can lead to an infection of the sinus. The inflamed state that results will cause facial pain and sometimes headaches.

The purpose of the poultices is to encourage the flow of wastes out of the sinuses, and send the pain with them. To treat the sinuses it is necessary to use several poultices in rotation, with one poultice replacing another as soon as the first cools, because poultices only stimulate the flow of phlegm when they are hot. Three poultices are therefore necessary to treat the frontal sinus, and three more to treat the maxillary sinus (if all sinuses are afflicted).

Flax Meal Poultice

10 ounces of flax meal (found in natural food stores)

6 paper towels or handkerchiefs

1 spatula

2 thin pieces of cloth

1 wool cloth

1 pot with a lid, filled with boiling water, for
reheating the poultices

Preparation: Combine the flax meal with twice its volume of water and simmer until a very uniform paste has formed. Spread the paste over the center surface of the handkerchiefs or paper towels in a layer that is slightly less than a half inch thick. Make three poultices large enough to cover the frontal sinuses (the forehead, in other words) and three poultices to cover the maxillary sinuses (from the top of the left cheek, over the nose, and across the top of the right cheek). Fold the handkerchiefs or paper towels over the poultices so that the flax meal is completely sealed inside. Place two of each size poultice on a radiator or on top of the lid of a pot of boiling water to keep hot.

Application: Wrap each of the two remaining poultices in a thin cloth. Then, after testing their temperature on the inside of the forearm, place them over the sinuses. Cover them with the wool cloth so they retain their heat for as long as possible. When they cool to lukewarm, which will take several minutes, remove them and replace them with new poultices that were prepared earlier and are being kept hot. The poultices are therefore renewed by rotation; those that were just used are reheated while their replacements are in use.

Duration: Renew the poultices every few minutes for a total of thirty to sixty minutes.

Frequency: Repeat two or three times a day during the crisis period, or more if necessary.

🖐 Good to Know

Flax (*Linum usitatissimum*): This is a plant with pretty blue flowers that produces seeds with lots of mucilage. These seeds can be taken internally to treat constipation. Flax meal is also known for its ability to loosen inflamed tissues.

The Mouth

SWOLLEN LIP (FROM A BLOW OR INSECT BITE)

Swelling due to impact, or a blow, to the mouth can be treated with an ice cube poultice (see page 40). Because of their disinfectant and analgesic properties, onion poultices are called for when there is an insect bite or sting. This poultice can be followed by an ice cube poultice to treat the swelling.

☞ Good to Know

It is well known that onions have multiple virtues for cooking, but they are also quite useful in therapy. They have a powerful ability to dissolve and eliminate toxins, as well as the power to kill germs (antibacterial action).

Onion Poultice

1 onion

1 knife

Preparation: Cut a slice of raw onion.

Application: After removing the stinger if it is a bee sting, place the slice of onion on the sting site, directly on the skin, checking to be sure the onion is making solid contact with the skin.

Duration: Leave it in place for five to twenty minutes.

Frequency: Apply just once. Follow with an ice cube poultice (see following preparation).

Ice Cube Poultice

1 or 2 ice cubes

1 small ziplock bag

1 small cloth

Preparation: Place the ice cubes in the ziplock bag and seal it. Wrap it once or twice in the cloth in order to protect the skin from the extreme cold of the ice.

Application: Place the poultice on the lip and painful area.

Duration: Leave in place for five to fifteen minutes.

Frequency: One application is generally sufficient.

TOOTHACHE

A toothache is quite often caused by tooth decay. The pain is caused by inflammation of the nerves and dental pulp (connective tissue and cells located inside the tooth). Poultices and compresses cannot cure or repair tooth decay, but they can calm the inflammation and reduce the pain pending proper medical attention.

Essential Oil of Clove Compress

Clove essential oil

Sweet almond oil or olive oil

1 handkerchief

1 wool cloth

Preparation: Blend 10 drops of clove essential oil with one teaspoon of sweet almond oil or olive oil and pour this mixture onto a handkerchief that has been folded over four or five times.

Application: Place the compress over the jaw next to the painful area (therefore outside the mouth). Hold it in place with your hand or with the help of a piece of wool cloth to encourage the spread of the active principles of the clove by the heat.

Duration: Continue in this manner for ten to thirty minutes.

Frequency: Repeat as needed until the condition can be remedied.

Variation: The same compress can be prepared with lavender essential oil or mint essential oil.

☝ Good to Know

Cloves (*Eugenia caryophilliata*) are well known for their powerful analgesic and antiseptic properties on the teeth and nerves.

Cabbage Poultice

Cabbage will not act as rapidly as clove and other essential oils to alleviate pain. See page 68 for instructions, which should be adapted for application to the jaw.

TOOTH ABSCESS

A tooth abscess is a pocket of pus caused by bacterial infection inside a tooth's inner "pulp chamber" that has spread to the root tip or around the root. It produces a small, soft swelling on the gums, is quite painful, and can cause the jaw or face to swell. The purpose of the poultices is to help the body get rid of the pus and to soothe the pain while waiting for more extensive dental treatment.

Clay Poultice

Healing clay powder (bentonite)

Cold water

1 wooden or glass container

1 wooden spatula to mix the water and clay together

Preparation: Blend the equivalent of two cups of clay with water to form a moist but firm paste.

Application: Apply the clay paste directly on the skin over the painful part of the jaw (outside the mouth). It should be a scant half inch in thickness.

Duration: As it dries, the poultice will suck the wastes from the tissues. Leave the poultice on for around two hours and then replace it with a new poultice. With each new application, the thickness of the poultice is gradually increased, first to three-quarters of an inch, then a generous inch. The purpose of this is to intensify its healing action. If the poultice becomes very hot while it is in place and its presence seems intolerable, it will be because it is full of wastes. Take it off and replace it with a new, cool poultice. Throw out the used clay as you go because it will be saturated with toxins.

Frequency: Repeat the applications until the pain stops.

The Eye

BLACK EYE

A blow to the eye region draws an abnormal flow of blood and lymph, which colors the rim of the eye in spectacular fashion. In response to chemical changes in the composition of the blood, the color then turns from red to green and then yellow to purple. The dramatic appearance of the eye in these circumstances has no relationship to the seriousness of the harm, which is generally mild.

By causing the tissues to contract again and reactivating blood circulation, a compress of freezing cold water will prevent the tissues around the eye from absorbing too much blood. It will be much more effective if applied as soon as possible after the injury.

Ice Water Compress

1 bowl of cold water

Ice cubes

1 cloth folded several times to a size that can cover
the entire eye region

Preparation: Place the ice cubes in the bowl of cold water. When the water is sufficiently cold, soak the compress in it, then wring out most of the excess water.

Application: Place the cold compress over the injured eye.

Duration: Remove the compress before it becomes too warm. Re-soak the compress in the ice water and place it back over the eye.

Frequency: Repeat as many times as you wish.

INFLAMMATION
(IRRITATION AND ITCHING OF THE EYES)

This can be an inflammation of the eyelids (blepharitis) or of the protective tissue of the ocular globe (conjunctivitis), an infection of an eye follicle (sty), or even simple irritation caused by smoke, dust, or bright sunlight. There is one plant that is particularly indicated for treating this condition: eyebright. Eyebright (*Euphrasia officinalis*) possesses disinfectant and anti-inflammatory properties that are especially effective in the ocular region. In addition to its healing properties, eyebright can anesthetize inflamed mucous membranes.

Eyebright Compress

3 or 4 cotton cloths large enough to cover the eye

Infusion of 1 tablespoon eyebright in 1 cup
of hot water

1 filter

Preparation: Filter the herbal tea after letting it steep for ten minutes.

Application: When the tea has cooled to lukewarm, immerse the cotton cloth in the liquid until it has permeated the fabric. Wring it out moderately and place it over the eye region. Press it very lightly to ensure that it is making good contact with the skin.

Duration: Apply for five to ten minutes, then repeat for three to four applications in a row. Soak a new piece of cotton cloth in the herbal infusion for each new application.

Frequency: Apply once or twice a day, or as needed.

Herb Compresses

Other herbs that are kind to the eyes include chamomile, cornflower, and calendula. These herbs can be substituted in the eyebright compress recipe above or combined with eyebright.

The Ear
....

EARACHE

Earaches are caused by inflammations in the ear, which can be close to the surface or deep within the orifice. In some cases they are also accompanied by modest or copious discharges. These painful afflictions can be soothed by warm poultices. Poultices made from onions are particularly effective. This is because the volatile properties of onions can stimulate circulation and interaction in areas of the ear that are difficult to access.

Onion Poultice
....

2–3 onions

Paper towel

1 thin cloth

1 scarf

Preparation: Chop the onions and sauté them with a little oil in a frying pan until they are soft and hot. Make a poultice that is slightly larger than the surface of the ear, so you can be sure the entire region will be covered. To do this, spread the cooked onions over a paper towel and wrap them in it completely by folding over the edges of the paper towel. Then wrap the whole package inside a thin cloth.

Application: After you have tested the temperature of the poultice on the inside of your forearm, delicately spread it over the region of the affected ear. If the heat is too intense, insert another layer of cloth between the ear and the poultice. The poultice should then be held in position with the help of a scarf tied around the head.

Duration: The poultice should remain in place for as long as it stays warm and is providing relief.

Frequency: Repeat as desired.

Potato Poultice

7–8 potatoes

Paper towels

Adhesive tape

1 thin cloth

1 spatula or rolling pin

1 protective cloth

1 scarf

Preparation: Boil the potatoes, remove them from the water when done, and allow them to cool for around twelve minutes. Then place the potatoes on the paper towel(s) in such a way that they will cover a surface a bit larger than the ear. Wrap the potatoes in the paper toweling by folding over the free ends of the paper. Use adhesive tape to hold them together if necessary, but make sure to leave one side of the poultice perfectly smooth and free of tape. Wrap the poultice inside a thin cloth, then use a spatula or rolling pin to slightly mash the potatoes to make sure they are spread out evenly.

Application: After testing the temperature of the poultice on the inside of your forearm, put the poultice on the ear and cover it with the protective cloth. Keep it in place with the help of a scarf.

Duration: Apply for one hour or as long as it remains hot and its presence is enjoyable.

Frequency: Apply once or twice a day.

The Throat

ACUTE SORE THROAT (LARYNGITIS, PHARYNGITIS, TONSILLITIS)

The ailments we are dealing with here are common sore throats, and although painful and unpleasant to experience, they are basically harmless. These are not the same as a severe sore throat infection, such as strep throat, which can have very serious complications.

Lemon Poultice

Lemon poultices have a very strong antibacterial and anti-inflammatory effect and are therefore great decongestants.

✍ Good to Know

Laboratory studies have shown that lemon juice is a powerful antibacterial and antifungal agent. This is one reason its use is recommended when eating oysters and fish and for disinfecting water.

> 1 large organic lemon
> 1 knife
> 1 rolling pin or bottle
> 1 thin cloth or large handkerchief
> 1 protective cloth
> 1 scarf

Preparation: Cut the lemon into four large, thick slices—almost half an inch thick. Line them up together on half the surface of the thin cloth, then fold the other half on top of them. With the help of the rolling pin or bottle, lightly crush them until they soften and begin rendering their juice.

Application: Place the poultice over the neck (with two lemon rounds on either side). Place the protective cloth on top of it, and then tie everything in place with a scarf that will keep the throat and the poultice warm. The acidity of the lemon may cause slight irritation of the skin, with stinging sensations. If this is too uncomfortable, remove the poultice and try another kind.

Duration: Apply for twenty minutes to one hour.

Frequency: Apply one or two poultices a day.

Onion Poultice

Like lemon poultices, those made with onions have a strong antibacterial and anti-inflammatory effect.

> 5–6 onions
>
> 1 thin cloth or large handkerchief
>
> 1 protective cloth
>
> 1 scarf

Preparation: Chop the onions into small pieces and sauté them with a little oil in a frying pan until they are soft and hot. Spread them over the thin cloth and fold its free ends together to completely wrap the contents. Make the poultice large enough to cover the entire throat area up to the ears.

Application: After testing the heat of the poultice on the inside of your forearm, delicately spread it over the throat. Cover it with the protective cloth and hold everything in place with the help of the scarf.

Duration: The poultice should remain in place for as long as it stays warm.

Frequency: Apply twice a day or more if necessary.

The Nape of the Neck

CERVICAL VERTEBRA PAIN CAUSED BY THE JOINTS (ARTHRITIS, RHEUMATISM)

When wastes are deposited between vertebrae of the neck, they irritate them and hinder their interaction. The arthritic pains that result can be soothed by heat. It intensifies blood circulation in the nape of the neck and facilitates the draining and elimination of wastes that have manifested as a kind of grit in the joints. The supply of heat should be maintained long enough to bring about circulatory changes.

Hot Compress

1 cloth folded several times to the size necessary to
cover the nape and lateral surfaces of the neck

Boiling water

1 kitchen towel

1 protective cloth

1 hot water bottle

1 wool cloth

Preparation: Soak the folded cloth in the boiling water. Set it on the kitchen towel, fold the towel over it, and use the towel to wring it out. (Holding the ends, twist in opposite directions.)

Application: Once you have tested the temperature of the compress on the inside of your forearm, place it over the nape and lateral surfaces of the neck. Cover it with the protective cloth, then place the hot water bottle on top. Make sure that the nape of the neck is sufficiently covered to stay warm by placing a wool cloth over everything.

Duration: Leave the preparation in place for thirty minutes to an hour.

Frequency: Repeat the treatment once a day for several weeks or until the pain has ceased.

Fango Mud Poultice, Potato Poultice

Poultices made from volcanic fango mud (see page 51) or potatoes (see page 46) are other options for treating this condition. Both of these procedures have a long duration (one hour). They can be aided by placing a hot water bottle on top of the poultice.

STIFF NECK, A CRICK IN THE NECK

This is a painful and irritating inflammation of one or both of the two sternocleidomastoid muscles, which run from the mastoid bone (behind the ear) to the sternum. The pain is felt primarily in the nape of the neck. Mobility is restricted by the pain, which is precipitated with every movement. A stiff neck, or crick, is caused by making an awkward movement, an uncustomary effort (sports, gardening), long hours driving or hunched over a computer, or sudden application of cold to the nape of the neck. It can also appear when someone has slept in an awkward position. The supply of heat with compresses and poultices will relax the muscles, soothe the pain, and accelerate the healing process.

Fango Mud (Volcanic Earth) Poultice

Volcanic earth that has already been prepared as
 a compress (can be found in natural food stores
 and vitamin shops)
Boiling water
1 protective cloth
1 wool cloth

Preparation: Immerse the compress for twelve minutes in the boiling water so that it absorbs the heat and becomes flexible from soaking in the water.

Application: After you have tested the temperature of the poultice on the inside of your forearm, place it over the nape and lateral surfaces of the neck. Then cover it with the protective cloth. The wool cloth should then be placed over this to ensure the heat is maintained.

Duration: Keep in place for as long as the poultice is warm.

Frequency: Repeat as desired for relief.

✗ Tips and Tricks

Poultices of fango mud (which is highly mineralized) can be used several times; simply reheat as needed in boiling water. However, be sure to identify the source of the mud, as some volcanic fango has been found to be radioactive and thus not suitable for pregnant women, children, or those with a weak immune system.

The Chest
....

Poultices and compresses offer surefire help for encouraging the elimination of wastes that congest the respiratory passages.

ASTHMA

In cases of asthma characterized by strong congestion of the bronchial tubes by phlegm—and not asthma brought on as an allergic reaction—poultices made with mustard powder can provide some degree of relief and sometimes even bring the attack to a complete halt. Mustard contains irritating substances that are somewhat aggressive to the skin, causing it to react strongly. It becomes red and hot because it summons a large quantity of blood from the depths of the body to the surface. The lungs are suddenly relieved of a considerable quantity of wastes this way, making it easier for the patient to breathe.

Mustard Powder Poultice (Mustard Plaster)
....
2 tablespoons of mustard powder

4–8 tablespoons of flour

1 bowl

Hot water

1 fine cloth large enough to cover the chest twice

1 protective cloth

Petroleum jelly (Vaseline or similar)

Preparation: Put the mustard powder and the flour in the bowl and mix them. Progressively add hot water until you obtain a moist paste that is neither too firm nor too runny in consistency. Spread this paste on half of the fine cloth, over a surface large enough to cover the chest, then fold the second half of the cloth over the paste to cover it. To protect sensitive body parts, smear petroleum jelly over the nipples and navel (this applies to men, too).

Application: Place the poultice over the chest and cover it with the protective cloth. It is normal to feel a slight stinging and burning sensation. In the beginning, check to make sure that this burning sensation is just an impression and not actually a burn on the skin, which would appear as a bright red color and be forming blisters. If you see signs of a burn, take the poultice off at once and wash the chest with water to remove any remnants of the mustard powder.

Duration: Leave the preparation in place for two to ten minutes. The main thing is not how long the poultice lasts, but that it causes a decongestant reaction in the lungs, which can occur even with an application of short duration. Also be guided by the good or bad reactions of the patient being treated.

Frequency: Use occasionally to provide relief.

⚠ Caution!

There is always a slight risk and degree of uncertainty surrounding the use of poultices and compresses that contain mustard powder, as the skin of some individuals is quite sensitive to this intentionally aggressive application; care and caution must be observed. However, this intensity is necessary to quickly redirect the toxins and relieve the respiratory passages.

Tips and Tricks

A mustard powder poultice or compress has the same effect when applied to the back of the thoracic region (slightly below the shoulder blades).

Mustard Powder Compress
. . . .

Mustard powder

**1 thin cloth three times larger than the surface of
the chest**

1 container of hot water (around 122°F)

1 protective cloth

Preparation: Spread open the thin cloth. Sprinkle the mustard
powder on the center third of the cloth in a layer around
2 mm thick. Fold the outer thirds of the cloth over it and
fold over the ends to create a tightly sealed compress. Plunge
it into the container of hot water, making sure to keep the
compress completely flat so as to avoid the mustard powder
clumping in some places and leaving others bare.

Application: After you have tested the temperature on the
inner surface of your forearm, place the dampened compress over the chest. The side that has only one thickness
of cloth should be the side directly touching the skin. Next
place the protective cloth over it. Every two minutes check
the skin's condition by lifting a corner of the compress;
the skin should be redder than normal but not bright red,
and there should be no blisters. Also be guided by whether
the sensations the compress is causing are agreeable or
unpleasant.

Duration: Keep the preparation in place for three minutes to
half an hour, but with careful monitoring.

Frequency: Repeat occasionally for relief.

⚠ Caution!

Because the lungs are extremely sensitive to cold during the acute phase of bronchitis, the application of moist, cold compresses is an extremely delicate matter that should be left to professional health practitioners. Consequently, the recommended applications in this book are all hot and dry. Note: Great care should be taken to prevent the patient from getting chilled during the time the poultice or compress is being placed on the body or removed.

BRONCHITIS AND COUGHS

Bronchitis is an inflammation of the bronchial and bronchiole tubes, the canals through which air enters the lungs. These tubes become increasingly narrow the deeper they lie in the body.

Inflammation is accompanied by an infection and is characterized by an overload of mucus that obstructs the respiratory passages and makes breathing more difficult. The body tries to eliminate these wastes by coughing and expectorating. Coughing can also be a symptom of sore throats, bad colds, and so forth.

Beeswax Compress

1 beeswax compress
1 thin protective cloth
1 wool cloth
2 hot water bottles
1 blanket

✋ Good to Know

Beeswax reheats wonderfully and pleasantly. It has a soothing effect on inflammation and liquefies the phlegm that the body is trying to dispel. It calms coughs, and thanks to its pleasant fragrance, it relaxes and relieves the patient.

Prefabricated beeswax compresses are available in drugstores and natural food stores and simply need to be heated before being applied. They can also be manufactured at home by dipping a cloth two or three times in liquefied beeswax and letting it cool to room temperature between immersions.

Preparation: Fold the protective cloth and lay it over a hot water bottle. Place the beeswax compress on top of this, followed by the wool cloth and then the other hot water bottle. If you purchased this compress, leave it in its protective packaging. If the compress is homemade, wrap it in a piece of aluminum foil to prevent it from leaking into the surrounding pieces of cloth during this preparation time, which is intended to heat all the different materials.

Application: Twelve minutes should be sufficient for heating the cloth wraps and the compress. Remove the compress from its packaging and, after testing the temperature on the skin of your forearm, place it directly on the skin over the chest. Then place the protective cloth on top of it, followed by the woolen cloth and then, depending on the size of the chest, one or both of the hot water bottles. Cover everything with a blanket. The heat emitted by the hot water bottle will keep the wax flexible and warm, which guarantees good contact with the skin. This contact is essential for the compress to be effective. The heat also encourages the spread of the aromatic qualities of the beeswax.

Duration: The compress should be left on for as long as its presence is pleasant, which can be several hours or even all night.

Frequency: Repeat as desired.

Variation: A second beeswax compress can be applied simultaneously to the upper and middle back.

Hot Compresses with Lavender and Eucalyptus Essential Oils

Lavender or eucalyptus essential oil

Sweet almond oil or olive oil

1 thin protective cloth

1 wool cloth

1 hot water bottle

1 blanket

☝ Good to Know

Essential oils possess powerful antibacterial properties and are natural antibiotics. The essential oils of lavender and eucalyptus have the additional property of liquefying phlegm and encouraging expectoration. They also soothe coughs.

Preparation: Mix 10 to 15 drops of the essential oil you have selected with one tablespoon of sweet almond oil or olive oil.

Application: Quickly spread the blend over the entire surface of the chest. Cover with the protective cloth (to prevent stains) and the wool cloth. Next place a hot water bottle on top to supply the beneficial heat that will help distribute the active properties of the essential oils into the lungs through the skin. Cover with a blanket.

Duration: Application should continue for one to two hours.

Frequency: Repeat as desired.

Variation: An identical compress can be applied to the back at the same time.

Onion Poultice

A poultice made from onions is another option for treating this condition. See page 48 for instructions, which should be adapted for application to the chest.

The Breasts

BREAST ABRASIONS

Because of their softening and healing effect, as well as their high vitamin A content (vitamin A is highly beneficial for the skin), carrot poultices are always recommended for treating abrasions and for cracked and chapped skin.

Carrot Poultice

3 medium organic carrots

1 very fine grater (handheld or food processor
    attachment)

Sterilized compresses (available from drugstores)

1 protective cloth

1 wool cloth

Preparation: Wash the carrots and shred them very finely, then spread them over the sterilized compress. The size of the poultice should be adjusted to cover the region requiring treatment. Seal the poultice by folding over the free ends of the compress.

Application: Lay the poultice over the abrasion, making sure it makes very close contact with the entire skin surface. Cover it with the protective cloth and the wool cloth.

Duration: Keep it in place for thirty minutes.

Frequency: Repeat as desired.

MASTITIS

The mammary glands sometimes become inflamed during the nursing period. The breasts become sore and nursing is difficult. Poultices of small-curd cottage cheese or Greek yogurt are especially indicated in this case, as their action is gentle. They will relieve the inflammation, decongest the glands, and soothe pain.

Cottage Cheese Poultice

Small-curd cottage cheese or Greek yogurt, at
  room temperature
1 spatula
Sterilized compresses (available from pharmacies)
1 protective cloth
1 wool cloth

Preparation: Spread the cottage cheese or yogurt over the middle of a sterilized compress so that a zone slightly larger than the region to be treated is covered. The thickness of the poultice should be less than one-quarter inch. Fold the free edges of the compress over the cottage cheese so that it is wrapped entirely.

Application: Place the poultice over the inflamed breast, making sure it is packed flat against the surface. Then cover it with the protective cloth, followed by the wool cloth.

Duration: Keep the poultice in place for twenty minutes.

Frequency: Apply once or twice a day, or after each time the baby nurses, if necessary.

☞ Good to Know

A cottage cheese poultice can be made using small-curd cottage cheese (not large curd), Greek yogurt, farmer's cheese, or quark (séré), whichever you have on hand.

NURSING: INSUFFICIENT MILK

Medicinal plants such as fennel seeds, anise seeds, caraway seeds, and verbena leaves have long been used in folk medicine to facilitate and stimulate milk production for nursing mothers when such assistance proved necessary.

Fennel Compress

1 tablespoon of fennel seeds

2 cloths large enough when folded in half to each
    cover one breast

1 protective cloth

1 wool blanket

Preparation: Steep one tablespoon of fennel seeds in a pint of hot water for ten minutes. Soak the cloths in the infusion and then wring out the excess moisture.

Application: After testing the temperature on the inner surface of your forearm, place one compress on each breast and cover both with the protective cloth and then the wool blanket.

Duration: Leave the compresses on for as long as they remain warm (fifteen to thirty minutes).

Frequency: Repeat twice a day.

Other Herb Compresses

Caraway, anise, and verbena compresses are prepared and applied in the same way as the fennel compress described above.

NURSING: TO REDUCE AND HALT THE FLOW OF MILK

Medicinal plants such as sage, mint, parsley, and chervil are recommended to dry up milk production during the weaning stage.

Their application in compresses is exactly the same as that for compresses used for treating insufficient milk production.

The Abdomen

LIVER AND GALLBLADDER CONDITIONS

Heat is a great friend to the liver and gallbladder, so much so that the compresses used to treat the liver are always hot except for certain acute infections, such as the different types of hepatitis. Whether the ailment is hepatic weakness, liver intoxication, difficulty digesting fats, or a bilious attack, heat will always bring relief by stimulating the production and secretion of bile.

The liver is located in the upper right-hand side of the abdomen. The bulk of the liver is protected behind the rib cage. Despite this, it can easily be stimulated by hot compresses.

Steam Compress

1 cloth folded over three or four times to a size that
will allow it to cover the region of the liver

Boiling water

1 kitchen towel

1 bath towel

1 wool blanket

1 hot water bottle

Preparation: Soak the folded cloth in the boiling water. Set it on the kitchen towel, fold the towel over it, and use the towel to wring it out. (Holding the ends, twist in opposite directions.) Wrap the wrung-out compress in a single layer of the bath towel.

Application: After testing the temperature of the compress on the skin of your inner arm, place it on the area of the abdomen over the liver. Cover this with the hot water bottle and the wool blanket. The hot water bottle will maintain the proper amount of heat for the entire time of the application.

Duration: Maintain for thirty minutes to one hour.

Frequency: Repeat occasionally as needed, or daily as a basic liver cure.

STOMACH PAINS (NERVOUS STOMACH, INDIGESTION)

Pains and stomach cramps due to indigestion or to nervous tension can be relieved by a hot compress with a hot water bottle.

Steam Compress

A steam compress applied over the epigastric region (the upper middle section of the abdomen) for ten to thirty minutes will bring about a comforting and relaxing reaction. See the instructions on page 62.

The Intestines

CONSTIPATION

Although constipation is primarily dependent on diet, compresses can improve the intestinal transit by stimulating and retraining the peristaltic muscles. The fact that this application is cold forces the intestines to react, which "reawakens" and strengthens them.

Cold Abdominal Wrap

1 cloth long enough to wrap around the hips one
and one-half times (from the bottom ribs to the
hip joint)

Cold water (approximately 68°F)

1 protective cloth that is the same size as the cloth
used for the compress

1 bath towel that is slightly larger than the
protective cloth

1 wool blanket

Preparation: Spread the wool blanket and the bath towel out on a bed where the person will lie on his back. Soak the compress cloth in cold water, then wring it out forcefully.

Application: To prepare the body for the cold application, warm it by rubbing it with your hands. Then wrap the moist cloth around the abdomen in such a way that it covers the belly from the bottom of the rib cage to the top of the hip joint. It should be pressed tightly against the skin to prevent any air from getting in beneath it, which would make it harder for the body to restore warmth to this area. Then wrap the protective cloth around the abdomen in the same way. The person should lie down on his back on the bath towel and the wool blanket, which are then wrapped around him. In several minutes the compress will become lukewarm and then hot thanks to the inflow of blood to the region, which will have a positive effect on the intestines.

✚ That Little Bit Extra

If the compress does not quickly heat, the body's reaction can be helped by placing a hot water bottle over the belly.

Duration: Apply the cold compress for forty-five to ninety minutes.

Frequency: Wrap the area once a day over a period of several weeks.

Hot Abdominal Wrap

When the cold application is not tolerable or has no reheating effect (for example, in elderly people or those with low vitality), it can be replaced by a hot abdominal wrap. In this case the stimulation will not be as strong because the heat source is coming from outside, rather than inside, the body.

The hot abdominal wrap is prepared and applied in the same way as the cold one, but hot water is used and it has a shorter duration—fifteen to thirty minutes, the time it takes for the compress to become cold. See below for specific instructions.

DIARRHEA (INTESTINAL FLU)

The application of wraps cannot cure attacks of diarrhea. However, hot compresses can relieve the pain and cramping.

Hot Abdominal Wrap

1 cloth long enough to wrap around the hips one and one-half times (from the bottom ribs to the hip joint)

Hot water

1 bath towel to be used to wring out the compress

1 protective cloth that is the same size as the cloth used for the compress

1 bath towel that is slightly larger than the protective cloth

1 wool blanket

Preparation: Spread the wool blanket and the larger bath towel out on a bed where the person will lie on his back. Soak the compress in hot water. Set it on the smaller bath towel, fold the towel over it, and use the towel to wring it out forcefully. (Holding the ends, twist in opposite directions.)

Application: After testing the temperature of the wrap on your inner forearm, wrap it around the abdomen in such a way that it covers the belly from the bottom of the rib cage to the top of the hip joints. It must make complete contact with the skin. The protective cloth is then wrapped around it in the same way. Then the patient lies on his back on the bath towel and the wool blanket, which are then wrapped around the abdomen.

Duration: Keep the wrap on for fifteen to thirty minutes.

Frequency: Repeat as desired.

The Bladder

ANURIA (URINE RETENTION, DIFFICULTY URINATING)

Poor elimination of urine or difficulty urinating occurs when the urinary passages are blocked due to an inflammation or clogged by deposits of wastes that normally should have been evacuated with the urine. In these cases a poultice of cabbage or clay should be used to clear the urinary passages of wastes that are clogging them and to reduce the inflammation of the tissues. Spasms can also be a cause for urine retention, in which case an input of heat can relieve the spasm and allow urine to flow normally.

Hot Wet Compress

This should be used in the case of spasms.

> 1 cloth folded until it is just large enough to cover
>   the lower belly
> Boiling water
> 1 kitchen towel
> 1 protective cloth
> 1 hot water bottle
> 1 wool blanket

Preparation: Soak the folded cloth in the boiling water. Set it on the kitchen towel, fold the towel over it, and use the towel to wring it out slightly. (Holding the ends, twist in opposite directions.)

Application: After testing the temperature on the skin of the inner forearm, place the compress over the lower belly. Cover it with the protective cloth, then the hot water bottle, and finally the wool blanket.

Duration: Apply for one hour.

Frequency: Repeat as desired.

☝ Good to Know

When choosing a cabbage, savoy cabbage with its curly leaves is the best choice, as it is more tender and juicy than other types of cabbage, and thus more malleable. In addition, it is rich in antioxidants. However, if it's not available, other varieties of green cabbage are also suitable.

Cabbage Leaf Poultice

Organic savoy cabbage (or other green cabbage if
    savoy is not available)

1 knife

1 rolling pin or bottle

1 protective cloth

1 wool blanket

Preparation: Pull off some unblemished cabbage leaves and use a knife to remove the large veins so that the leaves lie completely flat. Tenderize the leaves and make them flexible by crushing them with a rolling pin or large bottle; this will allow them to adhere well to the skin.

Application: Cover the lower belly with two or three layers of cabbage leaves. Make sure they are sticking securely to the surface of the skin and to each other. Cover them with the protective cloth and then the wool blanket.

Duration: Apply for one to two hours. If the poultice becomes too hot and uncomfortable, it is because it has become saturated with wastes. Take it off and replace it with a new one.

Frequency: Repeat application of the poultice two or three times a day, for several days in a row, until normal urination has been restored. This poultice can also be left on overnight.

Clay Poultice

A poultice made from clay is another option for treating this condition. See page 76 for instructions, which should be adapted for application to the lower belly.

CYSTITIS

Cystitis is an infection of the urinary passages with inflammation of the mucous membranes and frequent painful, meager urinations. Poultices of onions or compresses with essential oils relieve the pain by reducing the inflamed state with their antibacterial properties.

Onion Poultice

5–6 onions

1 thin cloth

1 protective cloth

1 wool blanket

Preparation: Chop the onions fine and sauté them with a little oil in a frying pan until they are soft. With the help of the thin cloth, wrap the onions to make a poultice that is a scant half inch thick and large enough to cover the lower belly.

Application: After testing the temperature on the inside of your forearm, spread the poultice over the region of the lower belly. Cover it with the protective cloth and then the wool blanket.

Duration: The poultice should remain in place for as long as it stays warm and its presence is providing relief. Because the bladder is extremely sensitive to cold when it is inflamed, take special care to ensure the patient does not become chilled when the poultice is applied or removed, as well as during the time it is in place.

Frequency: Apply two or three poultices a day, as desired.

Lavender Essential Oil Compress

Lavender essential oil

1 tablespoon of sweet almond oil or olive oil

1 cloth folded three times to a size that is large
   enough to cover the lower belly

1 protective cloth

1 wool blanket

1 hot water bottle, if needed to warm the compress

Preparation: Dilute 20 drops of lavender essential oil in the tablespoon of sweet almond or olive oil. Heat the cloth to be used as a compress on an indirect source of heat, such as a hot water bottle or radiator.

Application: Spread the oil over the entire surface of the lower belly. Place the lukewarm compress over it, then cover it with the protective cloth and the wool cloth. Keep it warm. The heat of the compress will encourage the penetration of the essential oil into the bladder.

Duration: Apply for one hour.

Frequency: Repeat two or three times a day.

The Uterus

PAINFUL PERIODS (MENSTRUAL CRAMPS)

Menstrual pains are due to spasms of the uterine muscle causing it to press against nearby blood vessels, briefly cutting off the supply of oxygen to the uterus. They can also be due to a congested state. Both heat and chamomile have a decongestant and antispasmodic effect.

☝ Good to Know

Chamomile (*Anthemis nobilis*) is most often recommended for digestive problems, such as indigestion, gastritis, and ulcers. However, its anti-inflammatory, healing, antispasmodic, and analgesic properties are active not only in the digestive tract but throughout the entire body.

Hot Chamomile Compress

1 thin cloth folded over several times and large
    enough to cover the lower belly

An infusion of 1 tablespoon chamomile in 1 pint of
    boiling water

1 kitchen towel

1 protective cloth

1 wool blanket

Preparation: Soak the folded cloth in the chamomile infusion. Set it on the kitchen towel, fold the towel over it, and use the towel to wring it out tightly. (Holding the ends, twist in opposite directions.) The less liquid it contains, the longer it will stay warm.

Application: After testing the temperature on the inside of your forearm, lay it over the lower belly. Cover it with the protective cloth and then the wool blanket.

Duration: The compress should be left on for as long as it remains warm (fifteen to thirty minutes).

Frequency: Repeat as desired.

The Back

....

MUSCULAR PAIN IN THE BACK (LUMBAGO)

In contrast to vertebral pains caused by skeletal problems, lumbago pain involves muscles and tendons. The pain can erupt following a wrong movement, overexertion or making an unaccustomed effort, maintaining poor posture for too long a time, a blast of cold air, and so forth. Applying heat to the stricken area is essential for relaxing the muscles, reactivating circulation, and eliminating irritants (toxins).

Potato Poultice
....

    7–8 potatoes

    Paper towels

    Adhesive tape

    1 thin cloth

    1 spatula or rolling pin

    1 protective cloth

    1 wool blanket

Preparation: Boil the potatoes, remove them from the water when done, and let them cool for around twelve minutes. Then place them on the paper towel(s) in such a way that they will cover a surface slightly larger than the area to be treated. Wrap the potatoes in the paper toweling (several sheets may be required) by folding over the free ends of the paper. Use adhesive tape to hold them together if necessary, but make sure to leave one side of the poultice perfectly smooth and free of tape. Wrap the poultice inside the thin cloth, then use a spatula or rolling pin to slightly mash the potatoes and distribute them evenly.

Application: After testing the temperature of the poultice on the inside of your forearm, wrap it in the protective cloth and place it on the back. Then place the wool blanket over it.

Duration: Maintain for one hour or as long as it remains hot and its presence is enjoyable.

Frequency: Apply once or twice a day.

PAIN OF THE NERVES AND BACK (SCIATICA)

Sciatica is a painful inflammation of the sciatic nerve, which emerges from the spinal column at the level of the lumbar vertebrae and descends all the way down the back of the leg. Sciatica can be distinguished from other back pain (vertebral or muscular) by the fact that it originates in the back and radiates downward into the buttocks and legs. The pain is caused by a compression of the sciatic nerve between two vertebrae (slipped disc) or an inflammation of the nerve caused by metabolic wastes (toxins).

✂ Tips and Tricks

Applications to treat sciatica can be either hot or cold. Depending on the individual, one may be much more effective than the other. It is difficult to determine in advance which will work best, but the patient will quickly realize whether heat or cold is providing relief.

Saint John's Wort Oil Compress

Saint John's wort oil (available in natural food stores, herb shops, and some drugstores)

1 thin cloth large enough to cover the region once it has been folded over three times

1 wool blanket

1 hot water bottle

Preparation: Pour 20 to 30 drops of Saint John's wort oil onto the folded thin cloth.

Application: Lay the compress on top of the entire painful area. To keep the compress hot, cover it with the wool blanket and a hot water bottle.

Duration: Keep the compress on the afflicted area for one hour at minimum or all night.

Frequency: Repeat as many times as desired.

Ice Cube Poultice

Ice cubes

1 ziplock plastic bag

1 protective cloth

Preparation: To be effective, this poultice must be placed only on the painful area. Its surface can therefore be fairly small and the number of ice cubes can be reduced accordingly. Place the ice cubes (or even one ice cube) in the plastic bag, seal the bag, and wrap it once in the protective cloth.

Application: Place the poultice directly on the specific area that is painful.

Duration: Apply for one to two minutes at most.

Frequency: Repeat as needed, depending on how much relief is obtained.

VERTEBRAL BACK PAIN

Generally speaking, all pains in the area of the spinal column are due to a combination of two factors: an accumulation of wastes between the vertebrae, and inflammation of different elements of the joint (vertebra, intervertebral disc, tendon, and so on) caused by the aggressive nature of the toxins stagnating there.

In both cases treatment consists of increasing circulation in the spinal column by applying heat so that wastes are expelled, the inflammation can be soothed, and damaged tissues are given the opportunity to repair themselves.

Potato Poultice

A poultice made from hot potatoes is one option for treating this condition. See page 72 for specific instructions.

Fango Mud Poultice

Volcanic earth that has already been prepared as
   a compress (available in natural food stores and
   vitamin shops)
Boiling water
1 protective cloth
1 wool blanket

Preparation: Immerse the compress for twelve minutes in the boiling water so that it absorbs the heat and becomes flexible from soaking in the water.

Application: After testing the temperature of the poultice on the inside of your forearm, place it over the region of the back needing treatment. Then cover it with the protective cloth. The wool blanket should then be placed over this to ensure that the poultice stays hot.

Duration: Keep in place for as long as the poultice is hot.

Frequency: Apply once or twice a day.

✗ Tips and Tricks

Fango poultices can be reheated with boiling water and used several times.

☞ Good to Know

What is the difference between fango and clay? Clay is a soil with a high mineral content that holds water and becomes slippery and pasty when wet. This is the clay used for modeling or by potters. Fango is a mineral-rich mud of volcanic origin. Since some fango has been found to be radioactive, pregnant women, children, and those with a weak immune system should take care to identify the source of the mud.

Clay Poultice

Healing clay powder (bentonite)

Cold water

1 wooden or glass container

1 wooden spatula to mix the water and clay
   together

1 protective cloth

1 wool blanket

Preparation: Mix clay with cold water until it forms a paste. It should be moist yet firm in consistency.

Application: Apply the clay paste in a layer about one-half to three-quarters of an inch thick to the part of the back to be treated. Cover the poultice with the protective cloth and then the wool blanket. The body will heat the poultice.

Duration: Leave the poultice in place until it becomes completely dry.

Frequency: Apply once a day.

The Anal-Rectal Region

HEMORRHOIDS

Hemorrhoids are nothing but varicose veins affecting the anus. They can be inside or outside. The cold compresses recommended here to tone the relaxed tissues of the vessels involved are primarily active on external hemorrhoids.

Ice Cube Poultice

Ice cubes

1 ziplock plastic bag

Preparation: Fill the plastic bag with one or more ice cubes and seal it.

Application: Place the bag directly on the hemorrhoids.

Duration: Apply for five to fifteen minutes.

Frequency: Repeat as desired.

The Shoulder

MUSCULAR AND JOINT PAINS OF THE SHOULDER

Whether the pain is caused by osteoarthritis, sore muscles from intense exertion, or a wrong move, the beneficial warmth of hot compresses and poultices provides a general sense of relief while reducing pain and stimulating the healing process.

Hot Compress

1 piece of cloth folded over several times and large
enough to cover the shoulder

Boiling water

1 kitchen towel

1 protective cloth

1 wool cloth

Preparation: Soak the cloth in the boiling water. Set it on the kitchen towel, fold the towel over it, and use the towel to wring it out forcefully. (Holding the ends, twist in opposite directions.)

Application: After testing the compress temperature on the inside of your forearm, place it over the afflicted shoulder area and cover it with the protective cloth and then the wool cloth.

Duration: Keep the compress on for as long as it remains warm.

Frequency: Repeat as desired, even several times a day.

Potato Poultice

7–8 potatoes

Paper towels

Adhesive tape

1 thin cloth

1 spatula or rolling pin

1 protective cloth

1 wool scarf

1 wool blanket

Preparation: Boil the potatoes, remove them from the water when done, and let them cool for around twelve minutes.

Then place them on the paper towel(s) in such a way that they will cover a surface slightly larger than the area of the body requiring treatment. Wrap the potatoes in the paper toweling (several sheets may be necessary) by folding over the free ends of the paper. Use adhesive tape to hold them together if necessary, but make sure to leave one side of the poultice perfectly smooth and free of tape. Wrap the poultice inside a thin cloth, then slightly mash the potatoes (with the spatula or rolling pin) to spread them evenly.

Application: After testing the temperature of the poultice on the inside of your forearm, wrap it in the protective cloth and place it on the afflicted shoulder area. Keep it in place with the help of the wool scarf. Cover everything with the wool blanket.

Duration: Keep it on for one hour or as long as it remains hot and provides a pleasant sensation.

Frequency: Apply once or twice a day.

Volcanic Earth (Fango) Poultice

A poultice made from volcanic earth is another option for treating this condition. See page 75 for instructions, which should be adapted for application to the shoulder.

The Elbow

EPICONDYLITIS (TENNIS ELBOW)

This is a painful condition that affects the elbow and forearm after too much demand has been placed upon them (gardening, sports, and so on). Keeping the arm immobile reduces the pain, but movement reawakens the pain and makes it worse.

The inflammation of the tendons can be calmed with the help of a poultice made from flax meal or cottage cheese.

Flax Meal Poultice

10–11 ounces of flax meal (found in natural food
   stores)
Paper towels
1 spatula
1 thin cloth
1 rubber band
Staples
1 pot with a lid, filled with boiling water, for
   reheating the poultice

Preparation: Combine the flax meal with twice its volume of water and simmer until a very uniform paste has formed. Spread the paste over the center surface of the paper towels in a layer that is a scant half inch thick. Shape the paste into what is required to make a poultice large enough to wrap around the entire elbow. Fold over the edges of the paper towels so that the flax meal is completely sealed in the center.

Application: Wrap the poultice inside a thin cloth, and after testing the temperature on the inside of the forearm, wrap it around the elbow. It can be held in place with a rubber band and staples.

Duration: Keep the poultice on for as long as it remains warm.

Frequency: Repeat the application as much as you like by reheating the poultice on a hot radiator, on top of a lid on a pot of boiling water, or in a double boiler.

Cottage Cheese Poultice

A poultice made from small-curd cottage cheese or Greek yogurt is another option for treating this condition. See page 83 for instructions, which should be adapted for application to the elbow.

The Wrist

ARTHRITIS OF THE WRIST (INFLAMMATION)

Arthritis in the wrist is a painful inflammation of the joint. The wrist becomes stiff, swollen, and extremely sensitive to pressure and movement. Clay and cold compresses calm the inflammation and improve blood circulation, which allows for better elimination of the toxins that are clogging the joint.

Clay Poultice

Healing clay powder (bentonite)

Cold water

1 wooden or glass container

1 wooden spatula

1 protective cloth

1 rubber band

Staples

Preparation: Blend clay with cold water until it forms a moist paste. It should be firm in consistency, not runny. It is possible to buy clay that is already in this state.

Application: Apply this clay paste around the wrist and cover it with the protective cloth. The layer applied should be about one-half to three-quarters of an inch thick. Secure it in place with the rubber band and staples. The poultice will be heated by the body.

Duration: The poultice may be left on overnight or until it dries.

Frequency: Apply one to three times a day.

The Hand

ARTHRITIS IN THE FINGERS

Arthritis is a disorder that can attack any joint in the body, but the hands are its most common targets. The inflammation of the joints makes them more sensitive to pressure and can be quite painful. The fingers become stiff and swollen, which is particularly apparent in the morning. In fact, it requires a certain period of activity to bring the fingers out of their numb state.

☞ Good to Know

Arthritis can be acute or chronic. When arthritis is acute, the joints are hot, even burning, and the use of cold (such as in the clay and cottage cheese poultices) is indicated to bring down the inflammation. In chronic arthritis the opposite is true; the joints are cold. In this case heat (such as in the potato and onion poultices) is recommended to warm them and restore proper blood circulation.

Clay Poultice

Healing clay powder (bentonite)

Cold water

1 wooden or glass container

1 wooden spatula to blend the water with the clay

1 protective cloth

Preparation: Blend the clay with cold water until it forms a firm, moist paste.

Application: Apply a layer of clay that is about half an inch thick around the afflicted fingers. Cover it with the protective cloth.

Duration: Leave the poultice in place until it dries or overnight.

Frequency: Apply once a day.

Cottage Cheese Poultice

Small-curd cottage cheese or Greek yogurt, at
  room temperature

1 spatula

Paper towel

1 protective cloth

Preparation: Spread enough cottage cheese over the middle of the paper towel to wrap around the finger. The thickness of the poultice should be less than half an inch. Fold the free edges of the paper towel over the cottage cheese (or Greek yogurt) so that it is wrapped entirely.

Application: Place the poultice around the afflicted fingers and then cover all of them with the protective cloth.

Duration: Apply for twenty minutes.

Frequency: Apply once or twice a day.

Potato Poultice

2–3 potatoes

1 handkerchief, paper towel, or thin cloth

Adhesive tape

1 thin cloth

1 spatula

1 protective cloth

Preparation: Boil the potatoes, remove them from the water when done, and let them cool for around twelve minutes. Then place them on the handkerchief in such a way that they will cover a surface slightly larger than the region requiring treatment. Wrap the potatoes in the handkerchief by folding closed its free ends. Use adhesive tape to hold them together if necessary, but make sure to leave one side of the poultice entirely smooth and free of tape. Wrap the compress inside a thin cloth, then use a spatula to slightly mash the potatoes and spread them evenly.

Application: After testing the temperature of the poultice on the inside of your forearm, place it around the afflicted fingers and hold it in place with the protective cloth.

Duration: Maintain the poultice for an hour or as long as it remains hot and its presence is enjoyable.

Frequency: Apply once or twice a day.

Onion Poultice

2–3 onions

1 paper towel or thin cloth

1 protective cloth

Preparation: Chop the onions and sauté them with a little oil in a frying pan until they are soft and hot. Spread the cooked onions over the paper towel and fold over the edges of the paper towel to wrap them up completely.

Application: After testing the temperature of the poultice on the inside of your forearm, delicately spread the onion poultice around the arthritic fingers and secure it in place with the help of the protective cloth.

Duration: The poultice should remain in place for as long as it stays warm and its presence is providing relief.

Frequency: Apply once or twice a day.

NAIL INFECTION

A sting or a splinter beneath the fingernail will sometimes cause an infection with a formation of pus. Given that cleansing the wound is made difficult, if not impossible, by the presence of the fingernail, the most promising solution is a clay or cabbage poultice. Both have drawing properties and can extract poisons from tissues.

Cabbage Leaf Poultice

Organic savoy cabbage

1 knife

1 rolling pin or bottle

1 protective cloth

Preparation: Pull off some unblemished cabbage leaves and use a knife to remove the large veins so that the leaves lie completely flat. Tenderize the leaves and make them flexible by crushing them with a rolling pin or large bottle; this will allow them to adhere well to the skin.

Application: Cover the finger with five or six layers of cabbage leaves and hold them in place with the protective cloth.

Duration: Leave the poultice in place for one to two hours. If the poultice becomes too hot, remove it and replace it with a new one.

Frequency: Repeat the application of the poultices until the finger has been healed.

Clay Poultice, Flax Meal Poultice

Poultices made from clay or flax meal are other options for treating this condition. For clay, see page 83 for instructions. Repeat until the condition has healed. For flax meal, see page 80 for instructions, adapting for application to the finger.

PINCHED OR HIT FINGERS

Fingers that have been pinched in a door or hit with a hammer become quite painful, swell, and form a bruise. Ice poultices placed on them as soon as possible after the mishap will soothe the pain and prevent a large bruise from forming.

Ice Cube Poultice

Whole ice cubes or chips (use a hammer or a
   blender that chips ice)

1 ziplock plastic bag

1 protective cloth

Preparation: Place the ice cubes in the plastic bag and seal it. Wrap the poultice of ice in the protective cloth, which should be folded once or twice depending on the individual's sensitivity to cold.

Application: Place the poultice on the injured finger.

Duration: Apply for three to ten minutes.

Frequency: Repeat if necessary.

Arnica Compress

Arnica cream (from a natural food store, herb shop, or pharmacy)

1 thin cloth folded three or four times

1 protective cloth

Preparation: Generously smear the top surface of the folded thin cloth with the arnica cream.

Application: Place the compress on the finger, with the arnica cream directly on the skin, and keep it in place with the help of the protective cloth.

Duration: Keep the compress in place for two to three hours.

Frequency: Repeat as needed.

🖐 Good to Know

Arnica (*Arnica montana*) is a mountain plant that has long been recommended for external treatment of all kinds of physical trauma: contusions, sprains, and lacerations. It also accelerates interior blood flow (which is helpful for treating bruises).

WHITLOW (ABSCESS IN THE SOFT TISSUE)

Whitlow is an infection of the fingertips that manifests twelve to twenty-four hours after being pricked on a sharp object or stung by an insect. The pain can be quite sharp and persistent when the pus does not drain easily.

Two kinds of applications are possible: poultices made from cabbage leaves or clay to drain the pus from the wound or simple hot compresses to keep the wound open in order to allow the pus to flow freely.

Hot Compress

1 piece of cloth, folded over several times
1 washcloth
1 protective cloth
Boiling water

Preparation: Soak the folded cloth in the boiling water. Set it on the washcloth, fold the washcloth over it, and use the washcloth to wring it out slightly. (Holding the ends, twist in opposite directions.)

Application: After testing the temperature on the inside of your forearm, place the compress around the finger requiring treatment and keep it in place with the help of the protective cloth.

Duration: Keep the compress in place for fifteen minutes to half an hour.

Frequency: Repeat as often as possible until the infection has healed.

Clay Poultice or Cabbage Leaf Poultice

Poultices made from clay (see page 83) or cabbage leaves (see page 85) can also be used to treat this condition.

The Hip

ARTHRITIS IN THE HIP

Like all inflammation of the joints, arthritis in the hip is painful and hinders freedom of movement.

In the acute phases—when the hips are in pain and accompanied by burning sensations—cold compresses or poultices are indicated, as they will soothe the pain and reduce inflammation.

When the problem is chronic, you must resort to the opposite extreme of hot applications in order to bring heat to the joint. This will intensify tissue irrigation and, with it, the elimination of toxins.

Cold Water Compress

Cold water

1 cloth folded over several times and large enough to cover the hip joint area

1 protective cloth

1 wool blanket

Preparation: Soak the compress in cold water, then wring it almost dry.

Application: Place the compress over the inflamed hip, then cover it with the protective cloth and the wool blanket.

Duration: Leave the compress in place for as long as it has a soothing effect on the pain, which will depend on the initial temperature of the water and the body's reactivity.

Frequency: Repeat the application as frequently as it brings relief.

Mustard Powder Poultice

1 tablespoon of mustard powder

4 tablespoons of flour

1 bowl

Hot water

1 fine cloth large enough to cover the hip twice

1 protective cloth

1 wool blanket

Preparation: Put the mustard powder and the flour in the bowl and mix them. Progressively add hot water until you obtain a moist paste that is neither too firm nor too runny in consistency. Spread this paste on half of the fine cloth, over a surface large enough to cover the hip, then fold the second half of the cloth over the paste to cover it.

⚠ Caution!

Poultices made with powdered mustard are tricky to use and should be used only with great care. They can cause blisters and are contraindicated for individuals with sensitive skin.

Application: After testing the temperature of the compress on the inside of your forearm, place the compress over the hip and cover it with the protective cloth and then the wool blanket. It is normal to feel a slight stinging and burning sensation. In the beginning, check every two minutes to make sure this burning sensation is only a sensation and not actually a burn on the skin, which would be indicated by the skin becoming bright red and blisters starting to form. If you see signs of a burn, remove the poultice right away and thoroughly clean the hip area to remove all traces of mustard powder.

Duration: As long as it is not burning the skin, keep the poultice on for two to ten minutes. The important thing is not how long the poultice stays on but that it provokes a reaction in the skin. This reaction will draw blood to the surface and, with it, the toxins that are congested in the joint. The skin's reaction—the effect of the poultice—can last for several hours after the poultice has been taken off.

Frequency: Repeat every three or four days, or as soon as the skin recovers its ordinary color.

Fango Mud Poultice, Potato Poultice

Poultices made from fango mud (see page 94) or potatoes (see page 93) can also be used to treat this condition.

The Knees

ARTHRITIS

Acute, painful inflammation of the knee joint requires rest as well as cold compresses and poultices that will calm the inflammation.

Clay Poultice

Healing clay powder (bentonite)

Cold water

1 wooden or glass container

1 wooden spatula to mix the water and clay together

1 protective cloth

1 rubber band

Staples

? Did You Know?

Human beings are not the only living creatures to use clay as a poultice; animals—both tame and wild—have recourse to them as well. Deer and wild boar will smear clay over their injured hooves or roll in clay-rich muds when they are ill, and horse trainers know well the value of clay poultices for equine injuries.

Preparation: Mix the clay with cold water until it forms a moist yet firm paste.

Application: Apply a layer of the clay paste that is one-half to three-quarters of an inch thick around the knee. Cover the poultice with the protective cloth and secure it in place with staples and the rubber band.

Duration: Leave the poultice in place overnight or until it becomes completely dry.

Frequency: Apply once a day.

Cold Water Compress

Cold water

1 cloth folded over several times that is large enough
   to wrap around the knee one and one-half times

1 protective cloth

1 rubber band

Staples

Preparation: Soak the folded compress cloth in cold water and then wring out almost all the liquid.

Application: Place the compress around the knee, then surround it with the protective cloth. Keep the whole thing in place with the rubber band and staples.

Duration: Leave the compress in place for as long as it has a soothing effect on the pain, which will depend on the initial temperature of the water and the body's reactivity.

Frequency: Repeat the application as desired.

OSTEOARTHRITIS

Chronic rheumatic problems of the knee are best treated by hot poultices. By activating blood circulation in this area, they encourage the elimination of wastes that are overloading the joint and stimulate the regeneration of damaged tissues.

Potato Poultice

7–8 potatoes

Paper towels

Adhesive tape

1 thin cloth

1 spatula

1 protective cloth

1 wool cloth

Preparation: Boil the potatoes, remove them from the water when done, and let them cool for twelve minutes. Then place enough of them on paper towels (you may need several) to make a surface large enough to cover the region requiring treatment. Wrap the paper towels over the potatoes. Use adhesive tape to hold them together if necessary, but be sure to leave one side of the poultice entirely smooth and free of tape. Wrap the compress inside a thin cloth, then use a spatula to slightly mash the potatoes and spread them evenly.

Application: After testing the temperature of the poultice on the inside of your forearm, place it around the ailing knee and hold it in place with the protective cloth.

Duration: Keep the poultice in place for an hour or as long as it remains hot and its presence is enjoyable.

Frequency: Apply once or twice a day.

Fango Mud (Volcanic Earth) Poultice

Volcanic earth that has already been prepared as
    a compress (available in health food stores and
    vitamin shops)
Boiling water
1 protective cloth
1 wool cloth

Preparation: Immerse the compress in boiling water for twelve minutes so that it absorbs the heat and becomes flexible from soaking up the water.

Application: After you have tested the temperature of the poultice on the inside of your forearm, place it around the knee. Then cover it with the protective cloth. The wool cloth should then be placed over this to ensure that the poultice stays hot.

Duration: Keep in place for as long as the poultice is warm.

Frequency: Apply once or twice a day.

☞ Good to Know

Fango poultices can be reused several times by reheating them in the boiling water. Since some fango has been found to be radioactive, pregnant women, children, and those with a weak immune system should take care to identify the source of the mud.

Mustard Powder Poultice

A poultice made from mustard powder is also an option for treating this condition. See page 90 for instructions to adapt for application to the knee.

WATER ON THE KNEE

Synovial fluid is the liquid that lubricates the space separating the different bones of the joint. When the joint has been struck or is suffering from inflammation (rheumatism), an unhealthy amount of this fluid sometimes collects in the joint, causing the knee to swell.

Generally the excess fluid is aspirated from the knee using a needle and syringe, but the same objective can be achieved using the powerful suction properties of cabbage leaf and clay poultices.

Cabbage Leaf Poultice

Organic savoy cabbage

1 knife

1 rolling pin or bottle

1 protective cloth

1 rubber band

Staples

Preparation: Pull off some unblemished cabbage leaves and use a knife to remove the large veins so that the leaves will lie completely flat. Tenderize the leaves and make them flexible by crushing them with a rolling pin or large bottle; this will allow them to adhere well to the skin.

Application: Wrap the knee with five or six layers of cabbage leaves and cover it with the protective cloth. Keep the leaves and cloth in place with the rubber band and staples.

Duration: Leave the poultice in place for one to two hours, or overnight. If the poultice becomes too hot, remove it and replace it with a new one.

Frequency: Repeat two or three times a day, until the desired result has been achieved.

Clay Poultice

A poultice made from clay is another option for treating this condition. See page 91 for instructions.

The Calf

CRAMPS
(CHARLEY HORSE)

Cramps are involuntary and temporary contractions of a muscle or group of muscles. They are generally painful, and when they occur at night, they interrupt sleep. Better irrigation by the bloodstream and relaxation of the contracted muscles can be achieved with the help of hot compresses.

Hot Wet Compress

1 cloth folded over several times that is large
   enough to wrap the calf one and one-half times
   and also large enough to cover the area between
   the knee and ankle

Boiling water

1 kitchen towel

1 protective cloth

1 wool cloth

Preparation: Soak the folded compress cloth in the boiling water. Set it on the kitchen towel, fold the towel over it, and use the towel to wring it out forcefully. (Holding the ends, twist in opposite directions.)

Application: Once you have tested the temperature of the compress on the inside of your forearm, wrap it around the calf. Cover this with the protective cloth and then the wool cloth to ensure that the compress retains its heat.

Duration: Keep in place for as long as the compress remains hot and is pleasant to feel, fifteen to thirty minutes.

Frequency: Repeat as desired.

VARICOSE ULCERS

When there are a large number of varicose veins and blood circulation has been greatly compromised, the body will try to eliminate the toxins that are stagnating in the poorly irrigated tissues of the calves by creating an artificial exit: a varicose ulcer.

Because of their powerful cleansing and healing properties, two poultices are especially recommended for treating this condition: poultices made from cabbage leaves and poultices made from clay.

Cabbage Leaf Poultice

Organic savoy cabbage

1 knife

1 rolling pin or bottle

1 protective cloth

Preparation: Pull off some unblemished cabbage leaves and use a knife to remove the large veins so that the leaves lie completely flat. Tenderize the leaves and make them flexible by crushing them with a rolling pin or large bottle; this will allow them to adhere well to the skin.

Application: Cover the part of the leg to be treated with two to five layers of cabbage leaves. Make sure they are sticking securely to the surface of the skin and to each other. Cover them with the protective cloth, which will help keep the leaves in place.

Duration: Keep in place for two to three hours, or all night. If the poultice becomes too hot and uncomfortable, take it off and replace it with a fresh one.

Frequency: Apply once a day until the ulcer has been completely healed.

⚠ Caution!

Dr. Jean Valnet has written of several possible reactions to cabbage leaf poultices: In the case of leg ulcers, eczema, and torpid or infectious wounds, the application of cabbage leaves sometimes triggers the momentary flare-up of the festering discharge or the reoccurrence of somewhat sharp pains. These phenomena are evidence of the detoxifying effect and tissue regeneration brought about by the therapy. In these cases the person should adopt a rhythm of discontinuous applications of one to two hours, separated by intervals of six to twelve hours, for several days.

Clay Poultice

Healing clay powder (bentonite)

Cool water

1 wooden or glass container

1 wooden spatula to mix the water and clay together

1 piece of gauze

1 protective cloth

Preparation: Mix the clay with cool water until it forms a moist paste. It should be firm in consistency, not runny. Spread the clay on a properly sized piece of gauze in a layer that is a scant half inch thick.

Application: Apply the clay poultice to the area requiring treatment and wrap it in the protective cloth.

Duration: Leave in place for one to three hours, or overnight. If the poultice becomes too hot or otherwise uncomfortable, remove it and replace it with a fresh one.

Frequency: Repeat application of the poultices once a day until the ulcer has healed.

VARICOSE VEINS (POOR CIRCULATION)

When the pressure on the walls of the blood vessels becomes too great, they can swell and become twisted and misshapen. Because blood circulation has slowed, the legs will feel heavy and fatigued. Varicose veins can sometimes be painful.

Ice Water Compress

1 bowl of cold water

Ice cubes

1 cloth folded several times to a size large enough
   to wrap one and one-half times around the area
   of the leg requiring treatment

1 protective cloth

1 bath towel

Preparation: Place the ice cubes in the bowl of cold water. When the water is sufficiently cold, soak the compress in it, then wring out a little of the excess water.

Application: Spread the bath towel on the bed in the area of the region to be treated when the patient is supine. Place the compress soaked in ice water around the leg and cover it with the protective cloth. Have the patient lie down on the bed with the bath towel beneath the compress.

Duration: Remove the compress before it becomes too warm. Re-soak the compress in the ice water and wrap it back around the leg.

Frequency: Use once a day for several weeks or until relief is experienced.

Lukewarm Compress of Medicinal Plants

The use of lukewarm compresses encourages the penetration of the body by the active properties of the medicinal plants being used.

> 1 cloth folded several times to a size large enough to wrap one and one-half times around the area of the leg requiring treatment
>
> 1 strainer
>
> 1 protective cloth
>
> 1 bath towel
>
> 1 thermometer
>
> Your choice of one of the following:
> - Witch hazel: four teaspoons of leaves boiled for two minutes in one quart of water
> - Cypress: one handful of leaves steeped for ten minutes in one quart of hot water
> - Yarrow: one handful of flowering tops steeped for ten minutes in one quart of hot water

Preparation: Let the herbal tea cool to slightly below body temperature, filter it, and soak the compress in the liquid. Remove the compress and wring it out slightly.

Application: Place the bath towel on the bed where the legs will be when the patient is supine. Wrap the region to be treated with the compress and cover it with the protective cloth. Have the patient lie on the bed with the towel beneath the compress.

Duration: Keep in place for twenty minutes to half an hour.

Frequency: Apply once a day for several weeks.

The Ankle

SPRAIN

A sprain is a painful lesion of the ligaments that results from twisting the foot in an abnormal way. The ankle becomes swollen and sometimes a bruise appears. To prevent the ankle from becoming too swollen, compresses of ice water and arnica are used. They are most effective if they are applied soon after the accident occurs.

Ice Water Compress

1 bowl of cold water

Ice cubes

1 cloth folded several times to a size large enough
   to wrap around the injured ankle

1 protective cloth

Preparation: Place the ice cubes in the bowl of cold water. When the water is sufficiently cold, soak the compress in it, then wring it out.

Application: Place the cold compress around the ankle and cover it with the protective cloth.

Duration: Remove the compress before it becomes too warm. Re-soak the compress in the ice water and place it back on the ankle.

Frequency: Repeat the operation as many times you like during the first few hours, then move on to the arnica compress.

Arnica Compress

Arnica cream (from a natural food store, herb shop,
or pharmacy)

1 thin cloth folded over four times and large
enough to wrap the ankle

1 rubber band

Staples

Preparation: Generously smear the thin cloth with the arnica cream. This will be the top surface of the compress.

Application: Place the arnica side of the compress directly on the skin of the ankle, making sure it is smooth and there are no folds. Fix the poultice in place with the rubber band and staples, making the compress tight enough to gently compact the tissues.

Duration: Leave the compress on for a full twenty-four hours.

Frequency: Repeat with a fresh compress daily for seven to ten days, depending on the sprain.

The Foot

COLD FEET (POOR CIRCULATION IN THE EXTREMITIES)

When a person's feet feel cold all the time, it is because of poor circulation. Blood flow can be accelerated by using revulsive poultices based on mustard powder or onions.

These two procedures are also used to draw blood down from the head to the feet as a treatment for headaches or migraines.

Onion Poultice

4–5 onions

Paper towels

1 thin cloth

1 pair of wool socks

1 hot water bottle

Preparation: Chop the onions into small pieces and sauté them with a little oil in a frying pan until they are soft and hot. Make two poultices that are slightly larger than the soles of your feet by spreading the onions on paper towels. Fold the paper towels over the onions to wrap them up completely.

Application: After you have tested the temperature of the poultices on the inside of your forearm, apply them to the soles of both feet. Pull the socks over them to keep them in place. When the poultices begin to grow cold, reheat them with the hot water bottle.

Duration: Continue for one hour.

Frequency: Apply once a day, or more if necessary (for example, in the case of headaches).

Mustard Powder Poultice

2 tablespoons of mustard powder

4–8 tablespoons of flour

1 bowl

Hot water

2 fine cloths large enough to cover the feet twice

Wool socks

Preparation: Put the mustard powder and the flour in the bowl and mix them. Progressively add hot water until you obtain a moist paste that is neither too firm nor too runny in consistency. Spread this paste on half of each of the fine cloths, over a surface large enough to cover a foot, then fold the second half of each cloth over the paste to cover it.

Application: After testing the temperature of the compresses on the inside of your forearm, place them over the soles of the feet and pull the socks on over them to keep them in place. It is normal to feel a slight stinging and burning sensation. In the beginning, check every two minutes to make sure this burning sensation is only a sensation and not actually a burn on the skin, which would be indicated by the skin becoming bright red and starting to form blisters. If you see signs of a burn, remove the poultices right away and clean the feet with water to eliminate all traces of the mustard powder.

Duration: Apply for two to ten minutes.

Frequency: Repeat twice a week.

🖐 Good to Know

There is always a little risk and uncertainty when using mustard powder poultices, because some people's skin is more sensitive than others' to this intentionally more aggressive application. However, by proceeding cautiously and judiciously, it's possible to determine the patient's level of tolerance for this kind of poultice.

DEGENERATIVE OSTEOARTHRITIS OF THE FEET

Chronic afflictions of rheumatic origin should be treated with hot compresses in the context of a long cure. The heat has a beneficial effect by activating blood circulation and clearing out wastes that have accumulated in the joints.

Hot Compress

1 cloth folded over several times so that it ends up
   being slightly larger than the the foot
Boiling water
1 protective cloth
1 kitchen towel
1 wool cloth

Preparation: Soak the folded cloth in the boiling water. Set it on the kitchen towel, fold the towel over it, and use the towel to wring it out forcefully. (Holding the ends, twist in opposite directions.)

Application: Once you have tested the temperature of the compress on the inside of your forearm, place it around the foot and keep it in place with the protective cloth and the wool cloth.

Duration: Keep in place for fifteen to thirty minutes.

Frequency: Apply once a day during a long cure.

Potato Poultice

4–6 potatoes

Paper towels

Adhesive tape

1 thin cloth

1 wooden spatula

1 protective cloth

1 wool cloth

Preparation: Boil the potatoes, remove them from the water when done, and let them cool for around twelve minutes. Then place them on the paper towel(s) in such a way that they will cover a surface equivalent to the region requiring treatment. Wrap the potatoes in the paper toweling (several sheets may be required) by folding over the free ends of the paper. Use adhesive tape to hold them together if necessary, but make sure to leave one side of the poultice entirely smooth and free of tape. Wrap the poultice inside a thin cloth, then use a spatula to slightly mash the potatoes and spread them out evenly.

Application: After testing the temperature of the poultice on the inside of your forearm, wrap it around the foot and cover it with the protective cloth and wool cloth.

Duration: Maintain for one hour or as long as it remains hot and its presence is enjoyable.

Frequency: Apply once a day.

Fango Mud Poultice

A poultice made from volcanic fango mud is another option for treating this condition. See page 94 for instructions, applying the poultice to the foot.

GOUT AND ARTHRITIS IN THE TOES

Gout is an extremely painful affliction of the joints of the big toe, which becomes red and swollen when inflamed. The toe becomes so sensitive that even the pressure of a sheet or blanket is enough to provoke sharp pain.

The inflammation of the joint is due to an excess of uric acid that has been deposited there in the form of urates (uric acid crystals, known as a *tophi,* which is Latin for "stones").

The most recommended poultices are those of cabbage leaves and clay, because their drawing properties can suction the uric acid out of the tissues and thereby calm the inflammation.

Cabbage Leaf Poultice

Organic savoy cabbage

1 knife

1 rolling pin or bottle

1 thin protective cloth

Preparation: Tear off some unblemished cabbage leaves and use a knife to remove the large veins so that the leaves lie completely flat. Tenderize the leaves and make them flexible by crushing them with a rolling pin or large bottle; this will allow them to adhere well to the skin.

Application: Cover the toes with two or three layers of cabbage leaves and keep them in place with the thin protective cloth. Make sure they are sticking securely to the surface of the skin and to each other.

Duration: Apply for one to two hours.

Frequency: Apply once a day.

Clay Poultice

Healing clay powder (bentonite)

Cool water

1 wooden or glass container

1 wooden spatula to mix the water and clay
   together

1 thin protective cloth

Preparation: Mix the clay with cold water until it forms a moist yet firm paste.

Application: Apply a layer of clay paste to the affected toes and wrap the protective cloth around them. The layer applied should be a scant half inch thick.

Duration: Apply for one to two hours.

Frequency: Apply once a day.

WARTS AND CORNS

? Did You Know?

A wart is a soft growth on the body caused by a viral infection. A corn is a hard, painful growth that appears on the calloused layer of skin of the upper surface of the toes, caused by the skin being squeezed too tightly between the bone of the foot and the shoe.

These different tissue growths can be treated with small garlic poultices, which, because of their highly corrosive properties, will dissolve and destroy the excess tissue.

Garlic Poultice

1 garlic clove

1 knife

Adhesive bandages (Band-Aids or similar)

Preparation: Crush the garlic clove with the knife until it is a fine paste. To protect the healthy surrounding skin, place one or more adhesive bandages at the borders of the wart or corn.

Application: Spread the crushed garlic paste on the area requiring treatment and keep it in place with another adhesive bandage.

Duration: Leave the poultice on overnight.

Frequency: Apply one poultice a day for at least fifteen days.

✂ Tips and Tricks

A simpler approach is to simply rub the wart several times a day with a slice or chunk of garlic.

The Skin

BURN

Burns caused by contact with an open flame, a hot plate, an iron, and so on are treated differently depending on how soon they are treated. The immediate treatment consists of applying cold to the burn so that the skin loses the heat it has accumulated as quickly as possible. At this stage ice water compresses are indicated.

⚠ Caution!

Poultices and compresses are only indicated for superficial burns and not for second- and third-degree burns.

The purpose of the compresses and poultices after the initial burn period is still to cool the skin, but these are intended to help the skin regenerate as well.

Ice Water Compress

1 bowl of cold water

Ice cubes

1 cloth folded several times to a size large enough
to cover the burn

Preparation: Place the ice cubes in the bowl of cold water. When the water is sufficiently cold, soak the compress in it, then wring out some of the excess water.

Application: Place the soaked compress over the skin.

Duration: Before it becomes warm, remove the compress, re-soak it in the ice water, and lay it back over the burn.

Frequency: Repeat the applications as frequently as desired, until the pain ceases.

Carrot Poultice

Organic carrots

1 fine grater

1 protective cloth

Preparation: Wash the carrots and shred them very finely.

Application: Spread the carrots over the burn in a layer that is about one-quarter inch thick. Cover them with the protective cloth.

Duration: Leave the poultice in place for thirty to ninety minutes.

Frequency: Apply two or three poultices a day in the days immediately following the burn. After that, applications can be spaced out at greater intervals.

Cabbage Leaf Poultice

Organic savoy cabbage

1 knife

1 rolling pin or bottle

1 protective cloth *or* 1 rubber band and staples

Preparation: Pull off some unblemished cabbage leaves and use a knife to remove the large veins so that the leaves will lie completely flat. Tenderize the leaves and make them flexible by crushing them with a rolling pin or large bottle; this will allow them to adhere well to the skin.

Application: Cover the affected area with two or three layers of cabbage leaves and cover the leaves with the protective cloth. Make sure the leaves are in close contact with the skin and with each other. Hold them in place with the protective cloth or the rubber band and staples.

Duration: Maintain for one to two hours.

Frequency: Apply once a day.

ECZEMA

Eczema is a common skin ailment that appears as a more or less extensive patch of red skin covered by a scattering of blisters that break, then ooze, and ultimately form a scaly crust. Given the fact that the body is using the eczema as a means of ridding itself of toxins congesting its tissues, the poultices used to treat it should support these efforts of elimination, which can be achieved successfully with applications of clay, birch leaves, cabbage leaves, and flax meal.

📖 A Little History

Cabbage was used by the Romans for six centuries—both internally and externally—to cure all kinds of diseases. It was used as a purgative and for making poultices. Soldiers used cabbage to treat their wounds and regarded it as a panacea.

Clay Poultice

Healing clay powder (bentonite)

Cool water

1 wooden or glass container

1 wooden spatula to mix the water and clay together

1 protective cloth

Preparation: Mix the clay with cold water until it forms a moist yet firm paste.

Application: Apply a scant half-inch-thick layer of the clay paste to the affected skin surface and cover it with the protective cloth.

Duration: Leave in place for one to two hours.

Frequency: Apply once a day.

Birch Leaf Compress

Approximately three-quarter ounce of birch leaves (available at herb shops) steeped for ten minutes in 1 pint of hot water

1 thin piece of cloth folded over two or three times that is large enough to cover the area needing treatment

1 kitchen towel

1 protective cloth

1 hot water bottle

1 wool blanket

Preparation: Soak the compress cloth in the birch leaf tea. Set it on the kitchen towel, fold the towel over it, and use the towel to wring it out. (Holding the ends, twist in opposite directions.)

Application: After testing the compress temperature on the inside of the forearm, place it over the area needing treatment and place the protective cloth and hot water bottle on top of it. Once this is all in place, cover it with the wool blanket.

Duration: Keep in place for thirty minutes to one hour.

Frequency: Apply once a day.

🖐 Good to Know

Birch (*Betula alba*) is a good diuretic and also possesses sudorific, or sweat-inducing, properties. Its leaves are used in folk medicine to treat skin diseases.

Flax Meal Poultice, Cabbage Leaf Poultice

Poultices made from flax meal (see page 80) or cabbage leaf (see page 112) are other options for treating this condition.

FUNGAL INFECTION

In cases of fungal skin disease, the skin becomes red and starts to itch. It also starts peeling in little white pieces that leave a painful zone in their wake. Fungal infections are very common on the toes. The most effective compress for treating them is made with whey.

Whey Compress

Fresh whey, whey concentrate (for example, the
   Molkosan brand), or powdered whey*

Water

1 cloth for a compress

1 protective cloth

Preparation: If you're using whey concentrate, mix 1 table-spoon with 1 tablespoon of water. If you're using powdered whey, mix 3 tablespoons with 3–4 tablespoons of water. Fresh whey can be used undiluted.

Application: Soak the compress cloth in the whey and place it on the area that needs treatment. Be sure that it has close contact with the skin. Fix it in place with the protective cloth.

Duration: Leave in place for thirty to sixty minutes.

Frequency: Apply once or twice a day.

INSECT STING

The poison injected in an insect sting causes an inflammation reaction (welt) and itching. If the injected venom is very violent (such as bee venom), these sensations will be accompanied by pain.

With the help of a poultice you can obtain at least a partial neutralization of the poison, which will effectively reduce the inflammation, pain, and itching.

---

*Use powdered whey, *not* whey protein. Powdered whey has about 12 grams of protein content; whey protein supplements contain around 24 grams of protein.

Onion Poultice

1 onion

1 knife

Preparation: Cut a slice from the raw onion.

Application: Place the slice of onion on the sting site, directly on the skin, making sure the onion has solid contact with the skin.

Duration: Hold it on the sting for one to five minutes.

Frequency: One application is often sufficient.

Lavender Oil Compress

Lavender essential oil

1 small cloth

1 adhesive bandage (Band-Aid or similar)

Preparation: Fold the cloth over two or three times. Place 5 or 6 drops of the undiluted essential oil on it.

Application: Place the oiled side of the compress over the sting welt and keep it in place with the bandage.

Duration: Apply for one to two hours.

Frequency: Repeat two or three times a day, as needed.

🖐 Good to Know

The lavender plant (*Lavandula officinalis*), long used in traditional folk medicine, has analgesic, disinfectant, healing, and calming properties to treat all kinds of insect stings.

Clay Poultice

A poultice made from clay is another option for treating this condition. See page 81 for instructions.

ITCHING

There are a variety of compresses and poultices available to soothe the itching that accompanies certain skin disorders. The itching is due to irritation caused by the presence of toxins in the skin.

Hot Compress

1 piece of cloth folded over several times to a size
    that will cover the necessary area
Boiling water
1 kitchen towel

Preparation: Soak the folded cloth for the compress in boiling water. Set it on the kitchen towel, fold the towel over it, and use the towel to wring it out forcefully. (Holding both ends, twist in opposite directions.)

Application: Once you have tested the temperature of the compress on the inside of your forearm, place it over the irritated area. The hotter the compress, the more effective it will be.

Duration: When the compress becomes cool, renew it by soaking it again in the hot water.

Frequency: Repeat as many times as needed.

PIMPLES WITH PUS
(ABSCESS, BOIL)

Pimples with pus are sebaceous glands that are congested with toxins and have become infected. They are painful until they pop and allow the pus to flow out of them. Hot, wet poultices (such as flax meal) encourage the abscess to develop and eliminate the pus.

Flax Meal Poultice
Flax meal (sold in natural food stores)
1 facial tissue (Kleenex or similar)

Preparation: Combine the flax meal with twice its volume of water and simmer until a very uniform paste has formed.

Application: Let the cooked meal cool a little. After verifying that its temperature is tolerable for contact with the skin, spread a layer that is one-half to three-quarters of an inch thick on and around the pimple. Cover it with a facial tissue.

Duration: Leave it in place for as long as it stays warm (around thirty minutes).

Frequency: Repeated applications encourage the development and eruption of the abscess. To drain it, follow with poultices made from clay or cabbage leaves. See pages 113 and 112 for instructions.

SHINGLES

Shingles is a viral skin infection in which small blisters form over the affected area. As these blisters always form over the pathway of a sensitive nerve, the disease is quite painful. Very noticeable results can be obtained in this hard-to-treat disease by calling on a special blend of essential oils, including lavender, sage, thyme, eucalyptus, rosemary, and cypress.

Essential Oils Compress

Lavender, sage, thyme, eucalyptus, rosemary, and
   cypress essential oils
Cloth handkerchiefs
Sweet almond oil or olive oil
1 protective cloth *or* 1 elastic bandage
Staples

Preparation: Combine 2 drops of each of the essential oils listed above with 1 tablespoon of sweet almond oil or olive oil and mix well. The dosage can be higher or lower, depending on the sensitivity of the skin of the person in question. Fold several cloth handkerchiefs three or four times to obtain a surface large enough to cover the painful area.

Application: Generously soak the compresses with the oil blend and place them over the region afflicted by shingles. Secure them to the area with the protective cloth or an elastic bandage.

Duration: Leave in place for one to two hours.

Frequency: Repeat two or three times a day.

Cabbage Leaf Poultice

A poultice made from green cabbage leaves is another option for treating this condition. See page 112 for instructions.

SUNBURN

Overexposure to the sun will burn the skin, making it red, sensitive, and painful. A compress made from vinegar water or a cottage cheese poultice will refresh the skin and rapidly soothe inflammation and pain.

 Good to Know

Sunburn causes skin temperature to be higher than normal. Bringing the temperature down soothes the skin, especially since cold has anesthetizing properties.

Vinegar Water Compress

1 cup vinegar (any kind)

1 cup cool water

Bowl

1 cloth folded over several times with a surface large
   enough to cover the area requiring treatment

Preparation: Mix the vinegar and the cool water in a bowl. Soak the cloth in the mixture and lightly wring out some of the liquid.

Application: Place the cloth over the entire area that has been sunburned.

Duration: When the compress becomes hot, remove it and replace it with a cool one.

Frequency: Repeat as desired.

Cottage Cheese Poultice

Small-curd cottage cheese or Greek yogurt

1 spatula

Preparation: Spread the cottage cheese or Greek yogurt over the entire region that has been sunburned. The thickness of the poultice should be a quarter of an inch.

Duration: When the poultice becomes hot, remove it and replace it with a cool one.

Frequency: Repeat as desired.

General Disorders

ANXIETY, NERVOUS TENSION

Worries, resentment, and stress create a state of nervous tension that is sometimes difficult to control or moderate. A simple means of relaxing, releasing inner contractions, and calming anxiety is the use of ice on the solar plexus. After the initial phase in which the body must react to the low temperature of the compress, a second phase starts in which a surprising sense of serenity and well-being appears. Torso wraps can also provide a huge sense of relaxation.

Ice Cube Poultice

10–12 ice cubes

1 container of cold water

1 sponge cloth

1 protective cloth

1 blanket

Preparation: Undertake this procedure well away from mealtime. Immerse the sponge cloth in cold water and wring it out by twisting it tightly. Fold the cloth in half and place two rows of five or six ice cubes in the middle. Fold the edges of the cloth over to enclose the ice cubes.

Application: Place the smooth side of the poultice over the solar plexus, the depression in the belly just below the sternum (epigastric fossa). Cover it with the protective cloth and then the blanket. After several minutes the cold sensation will give way to a sensation of heat caused by the reaction of the body.

Duration: Keep in place for one to three hours.

Frequency: Repeat as desired.

FEVER

Fever is not an illness in and of itself. It is the result of an intensification of all the body's metabolisms when they are fighting against an invasion or infection. Interrupting a fever artificially constitutes actively working against the efforts the body is deploying to heal itself. It is only justified when the fever is too high or lasts too long and thereby exhausts the patient's strength or otherwise becomes dangerous.

The compresses and poultices used in the event of fever are not capable of stopping it, but they can reduce it. They are different depending on the results one is seeking to obtain.

When the fever hasn't manifested and the patient is cold and shivering, warm wraps are indicated. These will support the body's defenses and cause abundant perspiration, which will free the body of a large quantity of toxins.

When the fever is present and high in temperature (spiking), and bringing it down temporarily will protect the patient or provide a moment of rest, cold compresses need to be applied. These can be rather small (cold compresses of the calves) or quite large (wrap of the entire torso), depending on whether a major or minor effect is desired.

Hot Dry Wrap

1 sheet

2 wool blankets

2 hot water bottles

Preparation: Spread the two blankets out on the bed on top of one another. Spread the sheet on top of them.

Application: The patient should lie naked on top of the sheet with arms raised. Wrap the left side of the sheet around the chest and around the left leg. The patient's arms should then be lowered and stretched alongside the torso. Now wrap the upper right edge of the sheet around the chest (covering both arms) and the lower edge around the right leg. The wrap needs to be quite tight around the neck and feet in order to prevent any cold air from gaining entry. The edges of the wool blankets are then folded over the patient's body and hot water bottles placed on both sides of the torso.

Duration: The wrap should be left on until the patient is hot, which can take anywhere from forty-five minutes to two hours. Ordinarily the patient will begin sweating toward the end of the application.

Frequency: Repeat as needed.

Cold Compress with Vinegar on the Calves
(Vinegar Slippers)

1 pint of cold water

1 pint of vinegar

2 cloths folded over several times and large enough
   to each wrap around a calf one and one-half times

1 protective cloth

1 bath towel

Preparation: Spread the bath towel on the bed at the place
where the individual's calves will be when supine. Mix the
vinegar and water together. Soak the compresses in this
mixture, then wring them out slightly.

Application: Have the patient lie down on the bed on his back.
Place the compresses soaked in vinegar water around each of
the calves and then cover them with the protective cloth.

Duration: Remove the compresses after two to three minutes
and soak them again in the cold water. Repeat the application one to three times.

Frequency: Apply as needed.

Variation: Use cold water alone without any vinegar added.
The effect will be the same but not as intense.

👆 Good to Know

Vinegar socks or slippers are commonly used in folk medicine. They are one of the most effective methods for
extracting heat and bringing fever down in children.

Cold Torso Wrap

2 bath towels large enough to wrap around the
   torso one and one-half times

1 even larger bath towel

Cold water (around 68°F)

1 blanket

Safety pins

Preparation: Spread the large towel out on the bed to protect the mattress and bedding. Soak one bath towel in the cold water and wring it out slightly. The colder the water is, and the more water contained by the towel, the greater the heat loss will be. Determine the water temperature and the quantity of water in the compress based on the individual's level of vitality and resilience.

Application: With the person seated on the bed, naked, wrap the torso in the soaked towel, then wrap with the dry towel. If necessary, pin the towels together with safety pins to make sure the wrap holds up properly. The person should then lie supine on the bed and be covered by the blanket.

Duration: Continue until the wrap becomes hot, five to twenty minutes, depending on the fever.

Frequency: Apply one to three times a day, depending on what is needed.

INSOMNIA

Sleep can be facilitated greatly thanks to the use of compresses. Their calming and relaxing effects encourage people to fall asleep. Those with cold feet who are rather sensitive to the cold react well to warm compresses that supply the heat they need in order to relax. For others, cold compresses have a more soothing effect. Cold compresses on the calves draw blood from the top of the body to the bottom, slowing the mind. A relaxing effect is also triggered by the heat the body produces in reaction to the cold compress.

Steam Compress

1 cloth large enough to wrap around the torso one and one-half times

Boiling water

1 bath towel for wringing out the compress

1 protective cloth that is the same size as the wrap cloth

1 bath towel that is slightly larger than the wrap cloth

1 wool blanket

2 hot water bottles

Preparation: Spread the bath towel on the bed where the person will lie on his back. Soak the cloth for the wrap in the boiling water. Spread it on the bath towel reserved for wringing it out, and twist the ends of the bath towel in opposite directions to wring it.

Application: After testing the temperature on your inner forearm, wrap this wet cloth around the patient's torso. It should closely adhere to the skin. The protective cloth and the larger bath towel should be wrapped around the person in the same way. Once the person is supine, place the two hot water bottles on either side of the torso, then cover everything with the wool blanket.

Duration: Maintain for one to two hours.

Frequency: Repeat in the evening before going to bed, as part of a longer cure, or as needed.

Cold Compresses on the Calves

1 pint of cold water

2 cloths folded over several times and large enough
   to each wrap around a calf one and one-half times

1 protective cloth

1 bath towel

Preparation: Spread the bath towel on the bed at the place where the resting individual's calves will be. Soak the compresses in the cold water, then wring them out slightly.

Application: Place the compresses around each calf and then cover them with the protective cloth.

Duration: Remove the compresses once they have become warm.

Frequency: Repeat in the evening before going to bed, as part of a longer cure, or as needed.

Cold Torso Wrap

2 bath towels large enough to wrap around the
torso one and one-half times

1 even larger bath towel

Cold water (around 68°F)

2 hot water bottles

1 blanket

Safety pins

Preparation: Spread the large towel out on the bed to protect the mattress and bedding. Soak one bath towel in the cold water and wring out almost all the water. Determine the water temperature and the quantity of water in the compress based on the individual's level of vitality and resilience. To support the shock of contact with the cold water and trigger the reheating reaction, it is recommended that the individual be warmed beforehand by dry rubbing with the hands or by performing some physical exercises (e.g., squats or push-ups).

Application: With the person seated on the bed, naked, wrap the torso with the soaked towel, then wrap with the dry towel. If necessary, pin the towels together with safety pins to make sure the wrap holds up properly. The person should then lie down on the bed and is kept warm with the help of the hot water bottles placed alongside the torso and the blanket placed over him. The wrap, which starts cold, should gradually become warmer. If it does not become warm in the fifteen minutes following the start of the operation, it should be removed and the patient warmed back up by other means. Take the same steps if the patient begins to feel cold during the course of the application.

Duration: The wrap should be left on until the patient starts feeling relaxed or at the very least until it becomes warm.

Frequency: Repeat in the evening before bedtime.

Directory of Compresses and Poultices

COMPRESSES

POULTICES

WRAPS

Index

Page numbers in *italics* indicate illustrations.